Caring for Older People in the Community

Caring for Older People in the Community

Edited by Angela Hudson and
Lesley Moore

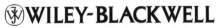

WILEY-BLACKWELL

A John Wiley & Sons, Ltd., Publication

This edition first published 2009
© John Wiley & Sons

Wiley-Blackwell is an imprint of John Wiley & Sons, formed by the merger of Wiley's global Scientific, Technical and Medical business with Blackwell Publishing.

Registered office
John Wiley & Sons Ltd, The Atrium, Southern Gate, Chichester, West Sussex, PO19 8SQ, United Kingdom

Editorial office
John Wiley & Sons Ltd, The Atrium, Southern Gate, Chichester, West Sussex, PO19 8SQ, United Kingdom

For details of our global editorial offices, for customer services and for information about how to apply for permission to reuse the copyright material in this book please see our website at www.wiley.com/wiley-blackwell.

Library of Congress Cataloging-in-Publication Data

Caring for older people in the community / edited by Angela Hudson and Lesley Moore.
p.   ;   cm.
Includes bibliographical references and index.
ISBN 978-0-470-51804-5 (pbk. : alk. paper)   1. Community health services for older people.   I. Hudson, Angela.   II. Moore, Lesley.
[DNLM: 1. Health Services for the Aged–Great Britain.   2. Aged–Great Britain.   3. Community Health Services–Great Britain.   4. Social Support–Great Britain.   WT 31 C2772 2009]
RA564.8.C373 2009
362.12084′6–dc22
2008044730

A catalogue record for this book is available from the British Library.

Set in 10 on 12 pt Sabon by SNP Best-set Typesetter Ltd., Hong Kong
Printed and bound in Singapore by Fabulous Printers Pte Ltd

1   2009

Contents

Contributors

Grace Boddy, RN, RHV, BSc (Hons) Soc Sci, PG Dip Health Promotion, Cert Ed (FE), Visiting Lecturer, Faculty of Health and Life Sciences, University of the West of England, Bristol. Grace's background was in health visiting before she joined nurse education. She has focused on sociology and social policy for nurses and other health care professionals.

Jane Buswell, MSc Health Studies, Dip Health and Social Care, RN, Nurse Consultant for Older People, University Hospitals Bristol NHS Foundation Trust, Bristol. Jane has specialised in the care of older people for many years in secondary care. She was a member of the national steering group developing the Let's Respect toolkit designed to help staff improve the way care is delivered to older people experiencing delirium, depression and dementia in the general hospital setting. As nurse consultant, she remains firmly grounded in clinical practice, with an emphasis on service delivery and practice development.

Tina Fear, MA, RN, Principal Lecturer, Faculty of Health and Life Sciences University of the West of England, Bristol. Tina's background is general nursing, health visiting and practice nursing. Her interests lie in the health and well-being of the older person, particularly the vulnerable, in terms of both care provision and prevention of abuse. She has a lead role in developing partnership working between care homes and other health and social care sectors, resulting in a regional Care Home Learning Network in the South West of England. She is currently involved in research projects involving care homes and other organisations.

Natalie Godfrey, RN, PGCE, Matron in Elderly Care, University Hospitals Bristol NHS Foundation Trust, Bristol. Natalie qualified in

1989, specialising in acute medicine for older people throughout her career. She has an interest in education and has been proactive in facilitating the professional development of clinical teams across the elderly care speciality. Natalie is currently undertaking an MSc in Advanced Practice.

Angela Hudson, MSc (Gerontology), PG Dip HE, BA (Hons) Open, RN, Senior Lecturer, Faculty of Health and Life Sciences, University of the West of England, Bristol. Angela's background is in working with older people in rehabilitation settings. Her interests lie with long-term conditions and their impact on the older person's health and well-being. She is the Professional Lead for Adult Nursing within the School of Health and Social Care. Angela has been involved in a number of projects including the facilitation of Action Learning Sets with four groups of community matrons. She is currently working with three local primary care trusts to deliver case management workshops.

Mary Marshall, OBE, Emeritus Professor, University of Stirling, Scotland. Mary Marshall has worked as a social worker with older people and as a researcher, campaigner, trainer and voluntary sector manager, and was, until 2005, the Director of the Dementia Services Development Centre at the University of Stirling. She now writes and lectures about dementia care.

Robin Means, PhD, MA (with CQSW) in Applied Social Studies, BA (Hons) in Social Administration, Professor of Health and Social Care and Associate Dean (Research and Knowledge Exchange), Faculty of Health and Life Sciences, University of the West of England, Bristol. Robin had a background in social work prior to moving to the University of Bristol in 1979, where he carried out a wide range of research projects on different policy and practice issues. He has a long-standing interest in both the history of welfare services for older people and the health and social care interface. He moved to the University of the West of England in 1998. He is an elected member of the Academy of Social Sciences.

Lesley Moore, MA, RN, Diploma of Nursing (Wales), Cert Ed (FE), RNT, Florence Nightingale Scholar, Fellow of the Higher Education Academy, Churchill Fellow, National Teaching Fellow, FRSA, Senior Lecturer Faculty of Health and Life Sciences, University of the West of England, Bristol. Lesley's background was in intensive care and recovery nursing for both the NHS and military sectors before becoming a clinical teacher and a nurse teacher. After majoring in social ethics, Lesley's research interests have focused on ethics and work-based learning. As an informal carer, she supported a close relative at home having renal haemodialysis. As a result of this experience, she is aware of the vulnerability of the older person with a long-term condition being cared for in the community during the transition of change in the NHS.

Kim Scarborough, RNLD, MSc (Profound Disabilities), PGCHE, PGC (Public Service Management), BSc (Hons) Community Studies, Senior Lecturer, Faculty of Health and Life Sciences, University of the West of England, Bristol. Kim's background is in learning disability nursing, with special interests in profound disabilities, care of older people and user empowerment. Kim is currently responsible for modules in both pre- and postregistration nursing awards and in developing learning opportunities for service users and carers. Kim is also a National Teaching Fellow.

Foreword

The publication of this book is well timed to stimulate debate and equip community nurses to respond effectively to the many challenges associated with caring for older people in community settings. Older people regard community nurses as their most important source of support in meeting their healthcare needs, with more than nine out of ten older people having contact with a community nurse each year.

Policy and practice in the care of older people in England has changed dramatically in the last 10 years, with wide ranging reforms to the healthcare system. There have been some major advances for older people. With a reduction in direct age discrimination, access to NHS treatment and services for older people has improved. Older people now account for 46% of NHS spending, a total of £41 billion in England, resulting in improved healthcare.

There has been a several-fold increase in the uptake of disease prevention services by older people, resulting in reduced death and disability resulting from heart disease, stroke and cancer. Furthermore, death from suicide among older people has dropped by about a third during this period.

The development of intermediate care services, although highly variable, has helped support recovery after an acute illness and reduced delayed discharge from hospital, benefiting about half a million older people each year in England.

Social services have targeted their home care services to those older people with the most intensive needs, so that over a third of older people requiring long-term care are able to continue to live in their own homes, up from a quarter 5 years ago. There has been a transformation in services for people with stroke, and a strong focus now on improving services for people with dementia, falls and fractures.

Best practice in end of life care, developed for people with cancer, has been successfully adapted for the care of older people, and is now widely deployed in older people's own homes, in hospitals and in care homes.

These achievements have been hard-won, because of pervasive myth and prejudice about older people in our society. There is a widespread and erroneous view that equates older people's care with social care rather than health, when the health spend is about five times that of social care.

Opportunities for treatment and prevention in healthcare are often downplayed in spite of research evidence which shows that, for many healthcare interventions, such as blood pressure control or hip replacement surgery, these are more cost-effective for improving health, independence and quality of life in older rather than younger people.

Simple but ineffective solutions are sometimes advocated for meeting the needs of older people with complex problems. For example, care coordination by case managers or community matrons is only effective when integrated into a multiagency response, underpinned by the principles of comprehensive multidisciplinary assessment and review. As much of the success of healthcare for older people is dependent on effective partnership working with social care, wider local government services and the independent sector, the frequency of organisational change in the NHS has disrupted the development of stable interorganisational relationships across these sectors.

Ministers in national government need to make their mark quickly, which creates pressure for new policy. The National Service Framework for Older People has provided some stability for policy implementation during a period when there have been five different Junior Ministers with policy responsibility for older people, five Health Secretaries and two Prime Ministers. Continuity in policy, for promoting health and well-being for older people, developing integrated systems of care and promoting culture change for securing dignity in care for older people, will be equally important in the years ahead.

A former Cabinet secretary advised me that, to be successful in national policy work, you need to keep your shape, like a 'cork in stormy seas'. I would advise all nurses working with older people in community settings to keep their shape, hold true to their values and their professional skills, but also be informed about the storms of policy and practice development that are blowing around them. This book will be of great value in helping you to withstand these pressures.

Professor Ian Philp
Professor of Health Care for Older People
Sheffield Institute for Studies on Ageing
University of Sheffield

Preface

It is hoped that this book will serve as a comprehensive resource for all nurses whose working life brings them into contact with older people and their carers in the community. The aim of the book is to provide nurses with the underpinning theoretical knowledge of sociological trends, increasing ethical issues and changing patterns of the population, in order to encourage them to understand the diversity of needs in the 21st century and the impact of modern technology.

Such challenges include the changing demographic pattern of the older population nationally and globally with the number of older people increasing; the fact that older people are living longer and utilising technology such as assistive devices to help maintain their health and well-being in the community, and the fact that new nursing roles are developing which will assist older people to remain independent at home. Each chapter will reflect these future perspectives.

In our current roles and past experience, we have gained expertise in the care of people with long-term conditions and in ethical dimensions. Angela has developed a profile that reflects care of older people and the challenges of managing long-term conditions, whereas Lesley as a Florence Nightingale scholar and ethicist, has developed an interest in autonomy, rights and end of life decision-making.

Angela Hudson
Lesley Moore

Introduction

This book is written with the intention of providing nurses with a comprehensive text that can be used to support practice work with older people. Care of the older person care is a speciality that on the surface gives the impression of undemanding care delivery, but encompasses complex physical, social and psychological needs. Nurses are one of the largest groups employed within the health service, and with older people as the biggest users of health and social care, it is imperative that nurses enhance their existing skills and knowledge to facilitate appropriately targeted care delivery to this client group.

The number of older people in the population is set to rise in the next 20 years as older people are living longer due to improved social conditions and technological advances. Caring for patients with diverse and complex care needs shifting from the acute to the community sector will pose many challenges. There will be an increased need for nurses to work within new boundaries and teams, undertaking new and differing roles. The user perspective will be increasingly important.

The book sets the scene by examining the past and current influences on practice, including the development of institutional care and the impact of demographic change in the older population. The influence of contemporary health and social care policy on older person care and practice is explored, and ethical tensions are examined. Section 2 focuses on contemporary challenges, including maintaining health and well-being and working with older people with a learning disability and with dementia. Section 3 explores future challenges, including the increasing use of technology, the role of the expert patient and new ways of working.

Throughout the book, the use of reflection points and scenarios will enable the student to reflect on current issues and consider how underpinning theory supports practice. Each chapter is evidence based and fully referenced, and contact details of relevant organisations will be included.

This book will help nurses meet the challenge of nursing and the ageing population with empathy and an understanding of diverse needs.

Section 1

Past and current influences on practice

Chapter 1
Historical perspectives from past to present

Robin Means

Introduction

This chapter provides an historical perspective for present debates about the need for health and social care to support older people to remain in the community wherever possible. It starts by looking at the main source of community support for older people, namely family and kinship, and explores how the role of the family has changed from pre-industrial Britain through to modern times. This leads on to a discussion of the changing role of institutions and how this has lead onto a growing emphasis on the importance of care in the community. The chapter goes on to set these debates within the attempts of Labour governments since 1997 to modernise health and social care services for older people. It is argued that the speed of change has generated significant tensions and problems 'on the ground', and hence that section is called 'Modernisation muddles'. The chapter concludes by pulling together the main themes of each section and drawing out from these the main implications for nurses and other healthcare professionals working with older people in modern Britain.

Family, kinship and older people

Older people in pre-industrial Britain

In *The Long History of Old Age*, Thane (2005) starts her edited collection by challenging a series of myths related to older people in pre-industrial society. At the core of these myths is the view that there were few older people in these societies since life expectancy was usually around only 40–45 years. Equally strongly held is the belief that the very few who did survive into later life were all cherished by their families and communities alike. She points out that the low life expectancy of this period was driven by very high death rates at birth and during infancy. The majority of those who lived through their childhoods did not go onto die in their 40 s but rather stood a very reasonable chance of reaching their 60 s and beyond. As a consequence, over 10% of the population in England was over 60 in the 18th century.

Many of these older people would have received great love and care from their immediate families. However, this was not true for all, for at least three reasons. First, labour migration in search of work was highly common in the pre-industrial period, which often resulted in older people being left behind:

> Separation of families because of the movement around the country or the world is not, as is often thought, a fact only of modern life. In the distant past people did not always live out their lives in one place; and when they left, in the days before mass communications and mass literacy, links with home and family might be lost for ever. (Thane 2005: 9)

Second, many couples lost all their children at birth and during childhood. Consequently, there were no adult children available to support them in later life. The third point relates to economic tensions between the generations in pre-industrial societies. Authors such as Stearns (1977) and Sarti (2002) have explored tensions relating to the transfer of wealth in employment areas such as farming. As Botelho (2005) argues, 'an aged parent's continued control over both house and estate left the adult son in a state of prolonged dependency, either unable to marry at all or placing both him and his spouse in submission' (p. 170).

Finally, veneration by the wider community was no more guaranteed than by the family. According to Thane (2005), old age per se did not generate respect but rather 'people of any age earned respect by their actions or because their wealth and power enforced deference' (p. 14). Poor older people were especially vulnerable – they might be looked after by their community, but equally they stood a strong chance of being largely ignored. Even those able to live with their children were likely to be dependent upon a household that was already in grinding poverty.

All of this raises the question of where these 'golden age' myths came from, especially in terms of this flawed belief in an organic community that cared for and respected all its older residents. Williams (1976) has claimed that 'community' is a crucial keyword in our society because of how it is used to explore major changes in culture and society. More specifically, he has traced how 'community' has been used from the 9th century BC to the 1970s as a mechanism to grieve for the passing of what is usually deemed to have been a much more organic and caring past. The biggest such fracture was caused by the Industrial Revolution, which encouraged a rather romantic view of community and family life in pre-industrial Britain.

Reflection points

- What would it have been like to be old and poor in pre-industrial Britain? What would be the differences from now? What would be the similarities?
- What would it have been like to be old and rich in pre-industrial Britain? What would be differences from now? What would be the similarities?

The impact of the Industrial Revolution

The late 18th and early 19th centuries saw massive changes transform Europe and North America through the combined impact of industrialisation, urbanisation and population growth (Cole and Edwards, 2005). The impact of all this on low-income older people was complex but often extremely negative. In many areas, although not all, it encouraged rural depopulation, with older people tending to be left behind to fend for themselves. Older factory workers were equally vulnerable when they 'lost their strength or became infirm or chronically ill and . . . could no longer keep up with the pace of the machine and the length of the working day' (Cole and Edwards 2005: 212). What happened to older people in such situations? One option was family support, but this was no less problematic in the 19th century than it had been in the previous two centuries. Younger kin may have migrated or been overwhelmed by responsibilities to their own children. As a result, such older people tended to try to stay at least on the margins of the labour market through part-time and casual work. Charles Booth, in his classic study of the *Aged Poor in England and Wales*, at the end of the 19th century found that 55% supported themselves through earnings and personal means, while 25% survived through a combination of earnings, parish provision, charities and support from relations (drawn from Cole and Edwards 2005: 236).

Such strategies were, of course, not an option for those whose severe health and frailty problems meant that it was impossible to remain even at the margins of the labour market. Many of these were supported by families as best they could, but others became dependent upon the Victorian Poor Law system. The 1834 Poor Law Amendment Act stated that the 'able-bodied' should only receive relief in the pauper's workhouse, whose regime needed to be sufficiently harsh and demeaning to encourage people to find work. In theory, this should have meant that older people with health problems could access either relief from the Poor Law parish from outside the workhouse or relief within it in a form that lacked the deterrent features of the regime being offered to the able-bodied.

The reality of the Victorian workhouse is open to debate, with many stressing the boredom and regimentation rather than the cruelty of workhouse life (Crowther 1981; Cole and Edwards 2005). What is clear is that many pauper inmates were older people who were either victims of unemployment or just too frail to work, even though defined as able-bodied. Even those defined as ill often experienced a lack of segregation with the 'able-bodied' and hence were effectively dealt with as if they were paupers (Cole and Edwards 2005).

However, this rather gloomy picture needs to be balanced against the emergence of growing numbers of middle class older people in the 19th century with access to considerable material resources well into late life. For example, the growth in home ownership fostered independence since 'homes, in addition to providing shelter and security for borrowing, can also be used to yield income from rent or taking in lodgers' (Cole and Edwards 2005: 221). Indeed, a small minority continued to retain control over considerable personal wealth and were likely to be surrounded by a wide circle of family, staff and friends. The experience of later life in Victorian Britain demonstrated massive inequalities.

Reflection points

- **Imagine life in a Victorian workhouse. Are there any similarities with life in a 21st-century care home?**

The family care of older people in the 20th century

So far, this chapter has warned caution about assuming that families were always available to support older people in the past. Nevertheless, families have always been a key support to older people in times of difficulty and one upon which government has always relied as a key mechanism to reduce health and social care costs falling on the state.

A series of classic studies in the late 1940s and 50s were able to evidence the extent to which many older people were embedded in family and kinship relationships. These included studies in Wolverhampton (Sheldon 1948), Bethnal Green (Townsend 1957; Young and Willmott 1957) and Woodford (Willmott and Young 1960). The Bethnal Green and

Wolverhampton research was in traditional working class communities, and findings emphasised the nature of reciprocity in kinship relationships. Grandparents, and especially grandmothers, were often taking on a caring role for grandchildren in order to support their children. In return, children, especially daughters, were frequently the key source of care and support for grandparents when their health declined. In Woodford, a middle-class outer suburb of London, geographical and social mobility had changed rather than loosened ties between grandparents and the next two generations. Hence, the main difference between Woodford and Bethnal Green was that:

> help from the older generation is less common in Woodford than help to them. The real contrast with the East End is that there the generations live side by side throughout life and at every stage kinship provides aid and support . . . In the suburb help is much more one-way, the younger couple . . . receiving much less than . . . they give to parents who are widowed, infirm or ailing. (Willmott and Young 1960: 72)

As these studies were completed in the mid 20th century, it needs to be asked whether family and kinship relations have further moved on with a much diminished caring role for families.

Chris Phillipson and colleagues from Keele University revisited Bethnal Green, Woodford and Wolverhampton in order to research this crucial issue (Phillipson et al. 2001). They found that most older people remained engaged with family-based networks, with spouses and daughters being especially crucial to the provision of emotional aid and a wide range of services. Overall, they felt able to argue that: 'The immediate family, then, offers an important protective role to older people: reassuring in times of crisis, playing the role of confidant and acting as the first port of call if help is needed in the home' (p. 251).

Against this, their results showed how most older people no longer defined themselves solely through their families. Friendships and leisure activities are now much more important, as also underlined by other researchers (Spencer and Pahl 2006). Many older people now have significant resources at their disposal, and not just the minority as in the 18th and 19th centuries. However, they stress how this is not true of all older people, with a minority lacking the resources to pursue such lifestyles and hence likely to feel especially isolated and vulnerable to social change.

Reflection points

- **What role did older relatives play in your own upbringing?**

The future of the caring family

Families, and the place of older people within them, continue to evolve and change. Harper (2006: 157) stresses the continued emergence of 'new family forms' such as 'reconstituted or recombinant stepfamilies, single parent families and cohabiting couples', who now constitute around 25% of Western European families. The extent of familial obligations to say, for example, an elderly stepmother who has been diagnosed with cancer is unclear, while low fertility rates means that an only child may end up trying to support not only two elderly parents but also two elderly step-parents (Finch 1989).

Overall, Harper stresses how households and family networks are becoming smaller, and she argues that this means that spouses will need to play a much stronger role in the future than in the past. The role of daughters is likely to diminish, especially in terms of availability for full-time care because of the increased likelihood of them being in full-time employment. More of the responsibility for care is likely to fall on partners rather than the next generation.

Hovering over all of this is the imminent move into retirement of the cohort that is often called the 'Baby Boomer generation', namely those born in the late 1940s and the 1950s. These individuals will initially represent an enormous resource to society; they will be important consumers (Gilleard and Higgs 2000, 2005), as well as having much to offer civic society through volunteering and other related activity. However, as they continue to age and their own health deteriorates, they will place considerable pressures upon both their families/step-families and upon the state in terms of health and social care expenditure.

The welfare state, older people and the changing role of institutions

The impact of the Second World War

Local authorities had taken over responsibilities for workhouses in 1929, and these were renamed Public Assistance Institutions (PAIs). However, many PAIs remained large cheerless buildings that a growing number of reformers felt were in desperate need of investment and change (Means and Smith 1998). One criticism was that they continued to contain large numbers of older workers unable to find employment and hence did not deserve the taint of pauperism. There was also concern about how the 1929 reforms had allowed Poor Law infirmaries to be transferred to the public health committees rather than the public assistance committees of local authorities. This did encourage such hospitals to improve the health-care on offer but often at the expense of being reluctant to admit older people with chronic health problems.

The resultant shortage of beds led to the development of very unsatis-factory conditions for older people in PAIs. Surveys in the 1940s presented the following picture:

> All are agreed that the reproach of the masses of undiagnosed and untreated cases of chronic type which litter our Public Assistance Insti-tutions must be removed? Without proper classification and investiga-tion, at present, young children and senile dements are 'banded together' in these institutions, along with many elderly patients whom earlier diagnosis and treatment might have enabled to return to their homes. (Nuffield Provincial Hospitals Trust 1946: 16)

In truth, such poor conditions had long been the norm, but it was only in the 1940s that reformers generated public and government concern. The reason for this seems to have been the impact of the Second World War.

The Second World War disrupted family and community support for all older people and not just those from poorer neighbourhoods (Means and Smith 1998). Older people needed to be evacuated from communities at risk from German bombing raids and they needed new accommodation when their homes were bomb damaged. However, perhaps even more importantly, support networks were undermined by sons being in the armed services and daughters increasingly involved in the war effort through such activities as working in the munitions factories. The ripple effect of this was even felt by middle- and upper-class households:

> The overriding claims of aircraft and munitions have swept the vast majority of maids, trained and untrained alike, into essential national war work. But total war has brought great sufferings and hardship to countless households: especially families which include the aged, the sick and young children. Family life among the middle and upper classes in this country has for generations rested largely on the assumption of domestic help of some kind being available. (Markham/Hancock Report 1945: 4)

The consequence of all this for better off older people was potentially dire, with some finding themselves in danger of becoming dependent upon PAIs, something which would have been unthinkable before the war.

In March 1943, the *Manchester Guardian* ran a story on a PAI visit to 'a frail, sensitive, refined old woman' of 84 years that was used to attack the regimentation of such institutions and the continued taint of pauperism:

But down each side of the ward were ten beds, facing one another . . .
On each chair sat an old woman in workhouse dress, upright unoccu-
pied . . . There were three exceptions to the upright old woman. None
were allowed to lie on their bed at any time throughout the day,
although breakfast is at 7am, but these three, unable any longer to
endure their physical and mental weariness, had crashed forward, face
downwards on to their immaculate bedspreads and were asleep. (Samson
1944: 47)

The clear implication was that such conditions might just about be
acceptable for working-class older people but certainly not for refined
(middle-class) ones. The article led to a campaign for the reform of PAIs
which the government agreed to tackle as part of post-war reconstruction.

Reflection points

- Imagine life as an older person during the Second World War. How well
do you think you would have managed?

Post-war reconstruction and services for older people

Overall, post-war construction went much further than just PAI reform
and covered the insurance and benefit proposals of the Beveridge Report
(1942), education, healthcare and social care (Glennerster 2007). In terms
of PAIs, the introduction of pensions, unemployment benefit, sickness
benefit and national assistance meant that older people should no longer
need to seek institutional care because of their inability to find employment in the labour market (Macnicol 2006). However, in terms of this
book and this chapter, the key change was the attempt to distinguish
between the healthcare and social care needs of these older people who
had previously all ended up in PAIs. Put crudely, the sick would be treated
through a National Health Service (NHS) established through the 1946
National Health Service Act and their services would be free. The frail
would be cared for in newly established Residential Care Homes under
the 1948 National Assistance Act, and this service would be charged for
by each pensioner paying 21 shillings a week from their new 26 shilling
state pension to the local authority.

The new NHS was in fact composed of three different elements: a hospital sector; an executive council sector responsible for GPs; and a residual

local authority sector that included district nursing, health visitors and midwives (this role was not taken away from local authorities until the implementation of the 1973 Health Services Reorganisation Act). In terms of hospitals, it remained true that the elderly chronic sick remained a low priority and hence a low-status medical specialism. Nevertheless, geriatric medicine pioneers such as Marjorie Warren, L.R. Cosin and Lord Amulree campaigned for improved care. All three were involved in a major British Medical Association review of geriatric medicine that was chaired by Dr Greg Anderson and that called for the following classification:

- The elderly
- The elderly and infirm
- The elderly sick
  - Senile sick
  - Long-term sick (potentially remediable)
  - Irremediable
- Elderly psychiatric patients
- Other special groups.

(Anderson Report 1947: 8)

The first group could manage in their own homes, while the elderly and infirm would either need family support or support through a Residential Care Home. The elderly sick could then be further classified so that active treatment and rehabilitation could be targeted at those most likely to gain from such input. Through such an approach, the elderly 'chronic sick' would no longer need to 'silt up' hospital provision.

As indicated, Residential Care Homes were established by the 1948 National Assistance Act. According to Nye Bevan, the Minister of Health:

the whole idea is that welfare authorities should provide them and charge an economic rent for them, so that any old persons who wish to go may go there in exactly the same way as many well-to-do people have been accustomed to go into residential hotels. (Quoted in Means and Smith 1998: 139).

Such aspirations were not realised in the late 1940s and 1950s. There was a shortage of building materials after the war so new smaller residential care homes were not built – instead there was a continued heavy reliance upon the old PAI buildings, often with the same 'Poor Law' staff who received no additional training. Such homes received a withering attack by Townsend (1964) in *The Last Refuge*. He found that 57% of accommodation was in rooms with at least 10 beds, and that the older institutions were in a state of shocking disrepair while some staff retained 'authoritarian attitudes inherited from Poor Law days' (p. 39). This situation was not tackled until the Residential Care Home building 'boom' of the late 1960s, at which point nearly all of these old PAIs were finally closed down.

The health and social care divide

However, of most relevance to this chapter is the divide that had been created between health and social care. The 1948 Act referred to people 'in need of care and attention' but did not define what this meant. What soon emerged was massive conflict between local authorities and NHS hospitals. Local authorities complained that the NHS had a shortage of hospital beds for elderly people requiring medical treatment, and that as a result they were ending up in Residential Care Homes despite needing much more than just 'care and attention'. Hospitals complained that their beds were being filled up with older people in need of care and attention rather than active medical treatment but were being told by local authorities that either there were no beds or that the elderly person in question was too frail for a care home (Means and Smith 1998).

Huws Jones (1952) spoke of how large numbers of elderly people were stranded 'in the no man's land between the Regional Hospital Board and the local welfare department – not ill enough for one, not well enough for the other' (p. 19). The response of government was to provide detailed guidance in 1957 on respective responsibilities for the 'partly sick and partly well'. Hospital authorities were told they were responsible for:

- Care of the chronic bedfast who may need little or no medical treatment but do require prolonged nursing care over months or years;
- Convalescent care of the elderly sick who have completed active treatment but who are not yet ready for discharge to their own homes or to welfare homes;
- Care of the senile confused or disturbed patients who are, owing to their mental condition, unfit to live a normal community life in a welfare home. (Quoted in Means and Smith 1998: 184)

Local authorities, on the other hand, were told that Residential Care Homes should provide:

- Care of the otherwise active resident in a welfare home during minor illness which may well involve a short period in bed;
- Care of the infirm (including the senile) who may need help in dressing, toilet etc, and may need to live on the ground floor because they cannot manage stairs and may spend part of the day in bed (or longer periods in bad weather);

- Care of those elderly persons in a welfare home who have to take to bed and are not expected to live more than a few weeks (or exceptionally months). (Quoted in Means and Smith 1998: 183).

What this guidance did was to effectively begin to define the term 'in need of care and attention' and to do this in a way that placed greater responsibilities upon local authorities than they had originally assumed to have been the case.

This guidance is now over 50 years old. However, governments have continued to struggle to provide definitive guidance on 'what is health-care?' and 'what is social care?', especially in the context of older people. Numerous further attempts have been made to tackle this issue 'for once and for all', but the boundary between the two has continued to shift, with local authorities being expected to provide services for older people at ever higher levels of dependency (Means et al. 2002). The Sutherland Report (1999) on long-term care was a Royal Commission set up by the incoming Labour government of 1997 to look at these issues yet again. The Majority Report of the Commission argued that no logical distinction could be made either between healthcare and social care or between those services which should be free and those which should be means-tested:

Older people need long term care not simply because they are old, but because their health has been undermined by a disabling disease such as Alzheimer's disease, other forms of dementia or a stroke. As yet these diseases cannot effectively be cured by medical care but people suffering from them will require ongoing therapeutic or personal care of different kinds in order to enable them to live with the disease. In this regard, the only difference between cancer and Alzheimer's disease is the limitation of medical science. (Sutherland Report 1999: 67)

As a result, the Majority Report called for free personal care, but this proposal was rejected by the government on the grounds of the high cost of making social care free rather than subject to means-testing.

Post-war reconstruction in health and welfare services for older people was focused primarily on institutions: the hospital for the sick and the Residential Care Home for the frail. By the 1960s and 70s, this focus came under increasing challenge. Governments were becoming concerned about the high cost of hospital care especially for older people, and this encouraged the start of the long process of arguing the case for more investment in community-based health and social care services, while a number of commentators were criticising poor conditions in not only Residential Care Homes, but also long-stay hospital provision (Means and Smith 1998). The next section looks at some of the reasons why it took so long to achieve a genuine shift to Care in the Community.

> **Reflection points**
>
> • Can you distinguish between what is healthcare and what is social care? What criteria are you using to do this?

Towards Care in the Community

The slow development of community health and social care services

At first glance, there would appear few obstacles to a major shift to Care in the Community for older people in terms of both community health services and social care. The first section stressed how the role of the family in elder care has long been emphasised. Annual reports of the Ministry of Health in the 1950s and 60s nearly all made reference to the need to keep older people in their own homes for as long as possible. The rationale for this was well expressed by Vaughan-Morgan et al. (1952) when they argued that at home 'they are surrounded by the things and people they know and love', while at home they are also 'required to help themselves in a hundred ways, all calculated to stimulate their physical and mental processes and so maintain their interest in life' (pp. 19, 20).

So what were the blockages? One of these was the limited powers of local authorities under the 1948 National Assistance Act. This enabled them to provide Residential Care Homes for those deemed to be 'in need of care and attention', but it gave no general powers to promote the welfare of older people through social work services, day care or visiting services, while Meals on Wheels services had to be supplied by a voluntary organisation rather than directly by a local authority. They could supply home help/home care through the 1946 National Health Services Act, but this was not made a mandatory duty until the early 1970s. District nursing and health visiting were provided by local authorities through the 1946 Act, but their priority tended to be children and young families rather than older people, while major co-ordination problems existed with regard to how these services related to GPs. Gradually, the legislative weaknesses of the 1948 and 1946 Acts were tackled, and most of the required changes were in place by the early 1970s. This was followed by 2 or 3 years of rapid service growth, but this was brought to a shuddering halt by massive oil price rises and consequent public expenditure cuts. The boom years of the welfare state were over without a full investment in community services ever having taken place.

But why did it take so long to get these changes into place, and why was there such an initial emphasis upon institutions? This chapter will now look at one important factor, namely concerns about the relationship of welfare reform to family care. Townsend explains this in the following forceful terms:

> The failure to shift the balance of health and welfare policy towards community care also has to be explained in relation to the function of institutions to regulate and confirm inequality in society and indeed to regulate deviation from the central social valued of self-help, domestic independence, personal thrift, willingness to work, productive effort and family care. (Townsend 1981: 22)

Put more crudely, families might abandon the care of their elderly relatives to the state if institutional care was of high quality or if community services were readily available.

The years after the main post-war reforms saw much talk of a 'slackening of the moral fibre of the family' (Thompson 1949: 250) and the need to challenge the view 'that the state ought to solve every inconvenient domestic situation', resulting in 'a snowball expansion on demands in the National Health (and welfare) Service' (Rudd 1958: pp. 348–9). Rudd was a consultant physician, and his message, and that of many others, was that the primary responsibility for the care of sick and frail elderly people lay with the family and that this must not be undermined by the welfare reforms of the 1940s.

The previous section outlined the classic community studies of Sheldon (1948), Townsend (1957), Young and Willmott (1957) and Wilmott and Young (1960). The picture that emerged from these was of the vibrancy of intergenerational family life rather than any slackening of moral fibre. This work was extended by Townsend when he explored *Old People in Three Industrial Societies* with international colleagues (Shanas et al. 1968) from a central concern to understand how support from the family intersected and meshed with support from the state. They concluded that health and welfare services do not conflict with family care: 'because either they tend to reach people who lack a family or whose family resources are slender, or they provide specialised services the family is not equipped or qualified to undertake' (Shanas et al. 1968: 129).

Gradually, governments began to see an expansion of community health and social care services as supporting the caring role of the family rather than undermining it.

Reflection points

- How would you balance the responsibilities of the state and the family in the care of older people?
- Did we get the balance right in the past? Have we got it right now?

Who should take the lead role in co-ordination?

The fact that community services were slow to develop did not stop endless debates occurring from the 1950s onwards about who should play the lead role in the co-ordination of such services. This has included numerous calls for both community health and social care services to all be under medical control rather than split between the NHS and local authorities. For example, the Gillie Report (1963) on *The Field of Work of the Family Doctor* claimed that the GP was 'the one member of the profession who can best mobilise and co-ordinate the health and welfare services in the interests of the individual in the community and of the community to the individual' (p. 9).

The restructuring of healthcare provision ushered in by the 1973 Health Service Reorganisation Act did take most healthcare functions away from local authorities but left them their social care or welfare functions. This left the GPs in a much stronger position to co-ordinate community health services on behalf of their patients, but in a very weak position with regard to social care input.

Indeed, by 1973, welfare services had been joined together with children's services and a range of other personal care services to create unified social services departments, which came into operation on 1st April 1971 as a result of the 1970 Local Authority Social Services Act. The 1970 and 1973 Acts had shown the continued belief in the need to distinguish between healthcare (GP, health visitor, district nurse, etc.) and social care (social work, home care, Meals on Wheels, etc.).

This resolution initially reduced pressure to establish a lead agency or profession across health and social care. The focus instead shifted to a range of mechanisms introduced by government to improve joint working across health and social services. The 1973 Health Service Reorganisation Act had established machinery for joint planning between health and local authorities through member-based Joint Consultative Committees. One of their main purposes was to plan for the rundown of long-stay hospitals and the encouragement of community-based services for a range of people including frail older people. Lack of progress led to the introduction of joint finance, a mechanism by which social services departments could, for a limited period, receive health authority funds to underpin community-based services for people leaving long-stay hospitals or to support people so as to avoid the need for future long-term NHS care (Means et al 2002: Ch. 5).

However, a key criticism of these types of initiative was that they involved relatively small amounts of money and hence impacted only at the margins of health and social care services. More specifically, the impact of joint care planning and joint finance was miniscule compared with the explosive growth of independent sector residential and nursing home care in the 1980s. This was initially funded through residents/patients being able to access social security benefits to pay for their care, and this enabled local authorities to close many of its residential care homes and hospitals to dramatically reduce its long-stay/continuing care beds. The scale of this growth was enormous. In 1979, 11,000 claimants in such homes were claiming only £10 million from the social security systems, yet by the early 1990s, 281,200 claimants were receiving £2.6 billion (Laing and Buisson 1994).

The Griffiths Review of community care and social services as the lead agency

Such developments were criticised not only because of the public expenditure consequences, but also because they were moving older people from one institution to another rather than supporting them to live in the community (Audit Commission 1986). There was also growing criticism of the continued failure to co-ordinate health and social care provision for older people (National Audit Office 1987). The then Conservative government invited Sir Roy Griffiths to carry out a review of the funding and organisation of community care.

Community Care: An Agenda for Action (Griffiths Report 1988) was widely expected to call either for social care services to move to health service control or for the establishment of a new organisation outside both the NHS and local authorities that would bring together community health and social care provision for the main community care groups, including older people. Instead, the review called for social services/local authorities to be given the lead agency role in community care, but to do this in a way that stimulated the provision of both care homes and social care services by the independent sector. The review also transferred responsibility for funding people in independent sector care homes to social services from the social security system, and hence effectively capped this major area of public expenditure.

These recommendations were to subsequently feed into the White Paper on *Caring for People* (Department of Health [DH] 1989) and then the 1990 National Health Service and Community Care Act, the community care elements of which were implemented on 1st April 1993. The White Paper set out the main responsibilities of social services as the lead agency; these included:

> Carrying out an appropriate assessment of an individual's need for social care (including residential and nursing home care), in collaboration as necessary with medical, nursing and other caring agencies, before deciding what services should be provided. (DH 1989: 17)

Such assessments were to be carried out by care managers who were likely to be, but not necessarily, social workers.

These reforms had not returned control of community health services such as district nursing to local authorities, but it had placed them in 'the driving seat' in terms of co-ordination at both the authority level (through community care plans) and at the level of the individual client (through care management). A crucial justification for these changes was that older people define their core needs in social rather than medical terms through their emphasis upon quality of life and retaining independence. However, would this new arrangement between health and social care last any longer than previous ones?

Long-term conditions and health as the lead agency

From the outset, it became clear that social services could attempt to influence health, but that it had few levers by which to encourage it to deliver healthcare in a way that integrated with its community care provision at both the strategic and individual levels. Not only this, but there was still no clear way forward for deciding 'what was healthcare?' and 'what was social care?' Health and social services continued to argue about who should supply what services for individual clients.

The 1990s, also, saw the issue of hospital discharge and bed-blocking emerge as a high-profile political issue. Increasingly, health blamed social services for these delays, a view that the Labour government of 1997 supported:

> On one day in September last year, 5,500 patients aged 75 and over were ready to be discharged but were still in an acute hospital bed: 23% awaiting assessment; 17% waiting for social services funding to go to a care home; 25% trying to find the right care home; and 6% waiting

for the right care home package to be organised . . . The 1948 fault line between health and social care has inhibited the development of services shaped around the needs of patients. (DH 2000: 29)

The quotation is taken from *The NHS Plan*, which expressed the desire to establish Care Trusts as 'new single multi-purpose legal bodies to commission and be responsible for all local health and social care' (p. 73).

Although a small number of Care Trusts for older people have emerged, these never took off as a popular way forward because of the legal and practical complexities in setting them up. Instead, the main thrust of government policy became strengthening the (lead) role of health, to the detriment of social services. More specifically, the focus has shifted to the long-term health conditions of older people rather than their social care needs. For example, *Supporting People with Long-term Conditions* (DH 2005) stressed the discomfort and stress experienced by the 17.5 million people with a long-term condition, but then focused down on how 5% of inpatients, most with long-term conditions, accounted for 42% of all acute bed days. The new model claimed to offer a new systematic approach to the care of patients with such conditions, with a view to significantly reducing the number of inpatient emergency beds. This is to be achieved through targeted health intervention via a new system of case management provided by experienced nurses who are to be called community matrons. The community matrons are:

likely to have caseloads of around 50–80 patients with the most complex needs and who require clinical intervention as well as care co-ordination. They will work across health and social care services and the voluntary sector, so that this group of patients received services that are integrated and complementary. (DH 2005: 16)

Healthcare provision now seems of more importance to government than social care, with the nurse as case manager replacing the social worker as care manager (Means et al. 2008: Ch. 5). Time will tell whether this arrangement proves any more robust than the community care reforms of the early 1990s.

Reflection points

- Should the nurse or the social worker take the lead in the care co-ordination for older people? How do you justify this view?

Modernisation muddles

The need to modernise public service has been a mantra for recent governments. The reasons for this are complex, but one influence has undoubtedly been a fundamental change in the general population in terms of the quality of services they expect to receive. Older people are no different in this respect. Earlier in the chapter, we looked at the future of the caring family in the 21st century. This will see the ageing of the 'Baby Boomer' generation who will expect to have a much greater say over their own healthcare than older people in the past. It is inevitable that healthcare systems will need to change in order to meet these increased expectations.

Few commentators would therefore argue the case for no healthcare reform at all. The real question is whether this desire for change has almost spun 'out of control' and hence become counterproductive. Within the space of this chapter, it is impossible to cover the sea of policy announcements, policy changes and organisational restructuring that has impacted upon health and social care under recent Labour governments. The 1997 government started by outlining broad modernisation plans for local authorities (Deputy Prime Minister 1998), social services (DH 1998) and health (DH 1997); and went on to embrace White Papers, National Service Frameworks and an almost endless stream of policy documents. In addition, there has been the growth of increasingly different policy frameworks in England, Scotland, Wales and Northern Ireland as a result of devolution. For example, Wales has free prescriptions but England and Scotland do not (although Scotland plans to implement free prescriptions from April 2011). Scotland has free personal care, England has rejected it, while Wales wishes to introduce it but cannot afford to do so.

In terms of health, England has seen among other things:

- the restructuring of health authorities and primary care trusts
- the emergence of foundation trusts
- the introduction of numerous milestones and targets
- the development of new approaches to commissioning and purchasing healthcare services
- fundamental changes in approaches to remuneration and workforce mixes
- a shift in emphasis to healthcare provision in the community rather than the hospital.

Equivalent changes in social care have included the break-up of social services departments into Children's Services and Adult Social Care

Services, the growing emphasis upon direct payments and personal budgets, as well as the same emphasis upon both milestones and workforce change.

The most coherent explanation of what the government is trying to achieve is probably to be found in *Our Health, Our Care, Our Say*, the White Paper on community services (DH 2006). A key thrust is that GP practices and primary care trusts would have a major focus on commissioning, with money increasingly following the patient, a process called practice-based commissioning. It is stressed in the White Paper that this requires close working with local authorities, especially if broader well-being and public health objectives are to be met. A cynic might conclude that the subsequent new *Commissioning Framework for Health and Wellbeing* (DH 2007) has many similarities with community care plans introduced as a result of the Griffiths Report (1988) (see above), but with health/primary care trusts rather than social care now very much in control. However, what is certain is that the health reform agenda of the government (and of the Conservative and Liberal Democrat parties) seems to guarantee a continued landscape of change at the levels of both policy and practice.

Means et al. (2008) argue that one consequence of all this change has been a growth in the gap between the formal objectives of policies and what is actually happening on the ground. They hence refer to 'modernisation muddles, in which managers and field-level staff struggle to keep pace with the demand for policy change and the ever increasing flood of directives, guidelines and indicators' (p. 250). This is a critical issue especially in terms of front-line staff since many older people will judge their healthcare in terms of how they are treated by those professionals with whom they have most contact. Nearly everyone enters a healthcare profession from positive motivations, but the impact of endless change and disruption can be a sense of feeling undervalued and hence the encouragement of what Lipsky (1980) called 'street level bureaucracy' (see also Hoggett et al. 2006). In other words, front-line staff end up offering the very opposite of person-centred care.

Reflection points

- Have you been affected by a major reorganisation at work, and if so, how did this affect you and your colleagues?

Conclusion

The noted historian Anne Digby (1989) has stressed that history does not respect itself precisely, 'yet, on a broader front, certain policy issues, dilemmas, problems and choices do recur in social welfare' and hence 'to forget the past record of these events is to force each generation to relearn what should already be known and thus make future developments less satisfactory than they might be' (p. 1). Hopefully, this chapter has supported Digby's perspective on the importance of historical perspectives on today's policy and practice dilemmas in the work of nurses and other health professions with older people.

The chapter concludes by drawing out three important themes. First, governments have always stressed the importance of family care for older people, and care in the community policy has usually been predicated upon the need to maintain the lead role of informal care rather than this being substituted by the state. Research evidence has consistently shown that children are committed to supporting their parents as their health declines, but that the nature of this changes as families themselves continue to evolve.

Second, governments have been continuously concerned about the high costs to the state of health and social care for older people despite the fact that older people have often been what used to be called 'a Cinderella service' in terms of their low priority for health and social care resources. This seems to often leave older people presented as some kind of threat or problem, especially to the health service, and also vulnerable to dependence upon poor quality services. Thus, the Boucher Report (1957) was based upon a 1954/55 survey of hospital and care home provision for older people and underpinned by concern around the high costs of hospital care for older people, while 50 years later policies on long-term conditions (DH 2005) seem to have been driven by exactly the same anxiety.

Finally, British provision for older people has been underpinned by this continued assertion that it is possible to make a distinction between free healthcare and means-tested social care services. It has been demonstrated how this health and social care boundary shifts over time, as do views about the respective roles of nurses and social workers, and of healthcare agencies and social care agencies. The present emphasis is upon the pivotal role of nurses/community matrons and supporting older people in the community. This places a major responsibility on nurses to try to ensure that these responsibilities are carried out in a way that supports older people to maintain their independence and social lives rather than just treating them in terms of their long-term illnesses.

References

Anderson Report (1947) *The Care and Treatment of the Elderly and Infirm*. London: British Medical Association.

Audit Commission (1986) *Making a Reality of Community Care*. London: HMSO.

Beveridge Report (1942) *Social Insurance and Allied Services*. London: HMSO.

Botelho, L. (2005) 'An idle youth makes a needy old age': the 17th century. In P. Thane (ed.) *The Long History of Old Age*. London: Thames and Hudson, pp. 113–74.

Boucher Report (1957) *Survey of Services Available to the Chronic Sick and Elderly, 1954–55*. London: HMSO.

Cole, T. and Edwards, C. (2005) 'Don't complain about old age': the 19th century. In P. Thane (ed.) *The Long History of Old Age*. London: Thames and Hudson, pp. 211–62.

Crowther, M. (1981) *The Workhouse System 1834–1929*. London: Batsford.

Department of Health (1989) *Caring for People: Community Care in the Next Decade and Beyond*. London: HMSO.

Department of Health (1997) *The New NHS: Modern, Dependable*. London: HMSO.

Department of Health (1998) *Modernising Social Services – Promoting Independence, Improving Protection, Raising Standards*. London: HMSO.

Department of Health (2000) *The NHS Plan: A Plan for Investment, A Plan for Reform*. London: HMSO.

Department of Health (2005) *Supporting People with Long-Term Conditions: An NHS and Social Care Model to Support Local Innovation and Interpretation*. London: Department of Health.

Department of Health (2006) *Our Health, Our Care, Our Say: A New Direction for Community Services*. London: HMSO.

Department of Health (2007) *Commissioning Framework for Health and Well-Being*. London: Department of Health.

Deputy Prime Minister (1998) *Modern Local Government: In Touch with the People*. London: HMSO.

Digby, A. (1989) *British Welfare Policy: Workhouse to Workfare*. London: Faber and Faber.

Finch, J. (1989) *Family Obligations and Social Change*. Cambridge: Polity Press.

Gilleard, C. and Higgs, P. (2000) *Cultures of Ageing: Self, Citizen and the Body*. Harlow: Prentice-Hall.

Gilleard, C. and Higgs, P. (2005) *Contexts of Ageing: Class, Cohort and Community*. Cambridge: Policy Press.

Gillie Report (1963) *The Field of Work of the Family Doctor*. London: HMSO.

Glennerster, H. (2007) *British Social Policy: 1945 to present*. Oxford: Blackwell Publishing.

Griffiths Report (1988) *Community Care: An Agenda for Action*. London: HMSO.

Harper, S. (2006) *Ageing Societies*. London: Hodder Education.

Hoggett, P., Mayo, M. and Miller, C. (2006) Private passions, the public good and public service reform. *Social Policy and Administration* 40(7): 37–56.

Huws Jones, R. (1952) Old people's welfare – successes and failures. *Social Services Quarterly* 26(1): 19–22.

Laing and Buisson (1994) *Care of Elderly People Market Survey*. London: Laing and Buisson.

Lipsky, M. (1980) *Street Level Bureaucracy*. New York: Russell Sage.

Macnicol, J. (2006) *Age Discrimination: An Historical and Contemporary Analysis*. Cambridge: Cambridge University Press.

Markham/Hancock Report (1945) *Report on Post-War Organisation of Private Domestic Employment*. London: HMSO.

Means, R. and Smith, R. (1998) *From Poor Law to Community Care: The Development of Welfare Services for Older People, 1939–1971*, 2nd edn. Bristol: Policy Press.

Means, R., Morbey, H. and Smith, R. (2002) *From Community Care to Market Care: The Development of Welfare Services for Older People*. Bristol: Policy Press.

Means, R., Richards, S. and Smith, R. (2008) *Community Care: Policy and Practice*, 4th edn. Basingstoke: Palgrave Macmillan.

National Audit Office (1987) *Community Care Developments*. London: HMSO.

Nuffield Provincial Hospitals Trust (1946) *The Hospital Surveys: The Doomsday Book of the Hospital Services*. Oxford: Oxford University Press.

Phillipson, C., Bernard, M., Phillips, J. and Ogg. J. (2001) *The Family and Community Life of Older People: Social Networks and Social Support in Three Urban Areas*. London Routledge.

Rudd, T. (1958) Basic problems in the social welfare of the elderly. *The Almoner* 10(10): 348–9.

Samson, E. (1944) *Old Age in the New World*. London: Pilot Press.

Sarti, R. (2002) *Europe at Home: Family and Material Culture, 1500–1800*. New Haven, CT: Yale University Press.

Shanas, E., Townsend, P., Wedderburn, D., Friis, H., Milhoj, P. and Stehouwer, J. (1968) *Old People in Three Industrial Societies*. London: Routledge and Kegan Paul.

Sheldon, S. (1948) *The Social Medicine of Old Age*. Oxford: Oxford University Press.

Spencer, L. and Pahl, R. (2006) *Rethinking Friendship: Hidden Solidarities Today*. Oxford and New Jersey: Princeton University Press.

Stearns, P. (1977) *Old Age in European Society, The Case of France*. New York: Holmes and Meier.

Sutherland Report (1999) *With Respect to Old Age: A Report by the Royal Commission on Long Term Care*. London: HMSO.

Thane, P. (2005) The age of old age. In P. Thane (ed.) *The Long History of Old Age*. London: Thames and Hudson, pp. 9–30.

Thompson, A. (1949) Problems of ageing and chronic sickness. *British Medical Journal* (30th July): 250.

Townsend, P. (1957) *The Family Life of Old People*. London: Routledge and Kegan Paul.

Townsend, P. (1964) *The Last Refuge: A Survey of Residential Institutions and Homes for the Aged in England and Wales*. London: Routledge and Kegan Paul.

Townsend, P. (1981) The structured dependency of the elderly: the creation of social policy in the twentieth century. *Ageing and Society* 1(1): 5–28.

Vaughan-Morgan, J. Maude, A. and Thompson, K. (1952) *The Care of Old People*. London: Conservative Political Centre.

Williams, R. (1976) *Keywords*. Glasgow: Fontana.

Willmott, P. and Young, M. (1960) *Family and Class in a London Suburb*. London: Routledge and Kegan Paul.

Young, M. and Willmott, P. (1957) *Family and Kinship in East London*. London: Routledge and Kegan Paul.

Chapter 2

Older people's experiences: social context and contemporary social policy

Tina Fear and Grace Boddy

Introduction

This chapter explores the social context of older people living in the UK, including demographic trends, quality of life and experience of ageism. Government policy is analysed, highlighting themes and impact on older people and their carers. Experiences of older people receiving services in all settings are described. Opportunities for reflection are provided throughout the chapter, to enable you to connect your own experiences to the topic under discussion.

Social context

Defining old age

Older people make up an increasing proportion of the population of the UK. The Office for National Statistics (2007) regard 'older people' as those over 50 years.

Reflection points

- How would you define 'old' or 'older' people? Does the age of retirement from work influence your view?
- Do you think that the individual's sense of well-being influences whether they feel 'old'?

Many sociologists would consider all age groups, including 'old age', to be socially constructed. Different societies view age and ageing in differing ways. In traditional societies, for example China and Japan, elders are seen to have wisdom and are accorded respect and authority within families and in society. Within industrialised societies, older people may be viewed as lacking the skills and abilities to contribute to modern working life due to advanced chronological age.

In a 'life-course' view of ageing, there are a series of stages that everyone passes through, characterised by roles and expectations of behaviours. In the 17th century, William Shakespeare identified 'seven ages of man' in his play *As You Like It*. The stages were infant, schoolboy, lover, soldier, justice, pantaloon (defined by the 2008 Oxford English Dictionary as a Venetian character in Italian commedia dell' arte represented as a foolish old man wearing pantaloons) and second childhood. Do these correspond with modern views of age? Age stages are understood and experienced in differing ways across history. Today's 'new' old bring their own ideas and experiences to older age. Individuals may challenge established views of norms of behaviour by doing things expected of one age category while chronologically belonging to another, for example people undertaking a 'gap year' for global travel as they approach old age or retire from paid work.

Changes to the ways in which older people think about themselves, together with improved experiences of health and incomes, result in the claim that 'fifty is the new thirty' (Roberts 2004). Groups such as the 'Baby Boomers', brought up in the anti-establishment 1960s, used to challenging the status quo and to being a powerful consumer group, may redefine both retirement and welfare provision in the future (Huber and Skidmore 2003).

It is important to recognise that older people are not a homogenous group. They differ in many ways, including chronological age, with new categories emerging of the young-old and old-old. Experience of life is likely to be different at 90 years from that at 50 or 70 years, although all will be regarded as older people. Gender, social class, ethnicity and disability may also contribute to differences in experiences of life and health and so will affect the individual's sense of well-being.

Inequalities in life and health

There is much evidence of the existence of inequalities in health (Acheson 1998). Differences in health-related personal behaviour and way of life may contribute to unequal experiences of health and disease. However, material deprivation, that is, poor socio-economic position characterised by low income and poor housing, is accepted as a major cause of health inequalities (Townsend and Davidson 1982; Acheson 1998). There is evidence that inequalities in health persist into older age as a consequence of inequalities experienced in childhood and adult life. A follow-up to the Whitehall study of health inequalities among various grades in the civil service demonstrated that people from lower occupational grades aged more quickly, with their physical health deteriorating more quickly than people in higher grades (Chandola et al 2007). Inequalities in health after retirement relate to social class and are associated with material and environmental disadvantage that has accumulated over the life course (Berney et al 2000).

Demography

How many older people are there in the UK today? The age composition of the population is changing, with a rising proportion of older people and a decreasing proportion of those under 16. A number of factors are involved in this, including falling fertility rates, falling infant mortality rates from the early 20th century with greater numbers surviving to adulthood, and, in recent decades, decreasing mortality rates at older ages (Office for National Statistics 2007). In the UK in 2003, 20 million people were aged over 50 (Office for National Statistics 2005), and this is expected to increase to over 27 million by 2031. In 2005, 16% of the population in England was over 65 years, and this is predicted to rise by 60% in the next 35 years. Under 16s made up 19% of the population in 2005, and this figure is falling. By 2014, the over 65s will exceed those under 16 for the first time (Office for National Statistics 2007).

The age composition of older people is changing too. People over 85 years formed 5.5% of those over 50 years in 2003, and by 2031 it will be 7.9 % (Office for National Statistics 2005). In 2004–05, those over 85 reached a record 1.2 million people, that is, 2% of the population. In 2007 more than 9000 people were over 100 years (Office for National Statistics 2007). Although the UK has an ageing population overall, ethnic minority populations are younger, with a small proportion of their populations over 50 years (Box 2.1). This is set to increase as immigrants from 1960s and 70s reach retirement.

Box 2.1 Percentage of ethnic minority groups aged over 65 years in the 2001 census (Office for National Statistics 2007)

- 11% Black Caribbean
- 2% Black African
- 7% Indian
- 4% Pakistani
- 3% Bangladeshi
- 5% Chinese

Reflection points

- **What implications might these population statistics have for health and social care services?**

There will probably be a falling percentage of younger people available to work and pay the taxes needed to provide pensions and formal care services for older people. Older people may therefore need to work to a greater age (Pensions Commission 2005). There could be an effect on the amount of services provided by the state, and older people may need to have made private provision for their own care. People providing informal care to family and friends may themselves be older (Wanless 2006). Consideration also needs to be given to providing appropriate support for people in minority ethnic groups (Mold et al. 2005).

However, the need for care is not determined by age itself, and older people have differing experiences of health, household circumstances, financial situations and family support networks that influence their needs. Morbidity compression theory (Jagger 2000) sees people entering retirement fitter and healthier than previous generations due to rising standards of living, healthier lifestyles and achievements in healthcare. It is proposed that this will mean a later onset of disability and a delayed progression of long-term conditions, so that morbidity will be compressed into a short period before death. A more pessimistic view is that the extended expectation of life also means an extended experience of disabling disease (Taylor and Field 2003). These differing views have different implications for the need for health and social care services.

Life expectancy is rising. In 2004–06, men aged 65 years could expect to live a further 16.9 years. Women could expect to live a further 19.7 years but to spend more years in poor health than men. There are also variations in life expectancy according to social class. In 2002–05, unskilled men could expect to live another 14.1 years and professional men 18.3 years. Unskilled women over 65 could expect 17.7 years and professional women 22 years (Office for National Statistics 2007). Women tend to live longer than men, and this is most marked among the very old, although improving male death rates are narrowing the gap. Whereas in 1951, in the over-50 age group, there were 77 men for every 100 women, in 2003 this ratio was 85 to 100. By 2031, it is projected that there will be 90 men per 100 women. Seventy-nine per cent of women over 85 are widowed compared with 6% aged 50–59 years. Older women are more likely to live alone or to be resident in a communal establishment than men (Office for National Statistics 2005).

Around 30% of households are headed by an older person, and over 60% of people over 85 years live alone. In 2005, 72% of people aged 65 and over owned their own homes, although some of these may be in poor condition (Department for Communities and Local Government 2006). Keeping warm is an important issue for older people. In 2005 in England and Wales, the deaths of 69 people aged 65 and over involved hypothermia as the underlying cause, according to their death certificates (Department of Health [DH] 2007a). The percentage of people living in nursing and residential homes was 4.5% in 2001, those over 90 years forming the greatest proportion of residents (Office for National Statistics 2005). It is important to consider the implications of these statistics for the quality of life for older people.

Quality of life

Reflection points

● **What factors are important in giving you a good quality of life?**

What do older people say is important for their quality of life? In an Economic and Social Research Council (2007) national survey of 999 people aged over 65 years, the issues described below were identified (Box 2.2). Half of the survey group said they had done most or all of what they had wanted to do in their life, two-thirds were optimistic in outlook, but one-fifth were less well off than they expected to be. About 10% felt they had little or no control over their lives. The most commonly reported fear of older age related to ill-health and reducing physical ability.

Box 2.2 Quality of life (Economic and Social Research Council 2007)

- Good social relationships with family friends and neighbours
- A good home
- A safe neighbourhood
- Good facilities and transport
- A positive outlook
- Psychological well-being
- Activities and hobbies
- Good health and functional ability
- Social roles and engaging in social and voluntary activities
- An adequate income
- Control over one's life

Research by Nazroo et al. (2003) with Black Caribbean, Asian Indian, Asian Pakistani and white older people found that similar quality of life factors were identified, but that white groups had the highest income, wealth and health scores, while Asian Pakistani people scored best for social support and perceived quality of local amenities. Racism was found to affect quality of life through discrimination in opportunities for promotion at work, which in turn affected income. Living in areas where racial crime and harassment occurred also affected quality of life.

Older people – subjective views of health

What do older people say about their health? Self-reported health findings of people over 65 years in the 2005 Health Survey for England (DH 2007a) found that more than half said their health was good or very good. Arthritis was the most common condition reported by women, and 65% of women reported difficulty in climbing a flight of 12 stairs without resting (compared with 48% of men). The most commonly reported disease for men (37%) was cardiovascular disease. A total of 23% of men and 29% of women had fallen in the previous 12 months. Almost two-thirds of people reported hypertension, and 22% had visited their doctor in the previous 2 weeks. Figures of 12% of women and 9% of men reported low levels of psychosocial well-being, resulting from a low level of happiness, depression and anxiety, sleep disturbance and reduced ability to cope.

Older ethnic minority populations have differing health problems related to ethnic group. In research with Caribbean, Indian, Pakistani and white groups, all ethnic minority groups had poorer health than the white group. Pakistani people had markedly poorer health than other minority ethnic groups. Pakistani men had the worst health, possibly due to their employment experience (Nazroo et al. 2003). In the UK census of 2001, 27% of all people aged 50–64 years reported a long-term limiting illness, but this increased to 54% among Bangladeshis, 49% in those of Pakistani origin and 20% of Chinese individuals.

Theorising old age

There are several different ways in which sociological theories attempt to explain older people's experience of life. A functionalist, disengagement theory would propose that, in the interests of equilibrium and stability in society, older people need to retire from paid work, supported by their pensions and savings, thus making way for younger generations (Giddens 2006). However, activity theory considers that older people can continue to be involved in society as grandparents within families and contributors to local community and voluntary organisations, as they gradually withdraw from society and prepare for death (Giddens 2006). Such roles may be rewarding but lack power and prestige in societies that value youthfulness. These views may also encourage government policy to use age to organise services for older people that separate and exclude them from mainstream provision (Victor 2005).

A political economy approach would emphasise the role of society in defining old age and the experience of being old. Patterns of employment and income in adult life influence experiences of older age, resulting in some people living in poverty while others, having financial security, are able to pursue their interests. In the UK, the state still influences the age of retirement from paid work. For many older people, leaving work makes them dependent on the state for income in the form of pensions and other benefits. Exclusion from paid work can lead to poverty and social exclusion, with women, disabled people and those from ethnic minorities being particularly adversely affected.

Ageism

As people grow older, they increasingly become aware of and experience ageism. Ageism is prejudice and discrimination on the grounds of age and could apply to a variety of age groups such as children, young and older people. Older people may be stereotyped or categorised according to assumptions about old age, for example that all older people are ill and have reduced mental capacity. This can produce prejorative or negative judgements such as seeing older people as no longer useful to society and creating a 'burden' on the welfare state. Such views can lead to discriminatory behaviour. Older people are seen as 'other', fundamentally different from ourselves, rather than ourselves in future years. Ageism is based in beliefs that originate in biological differences in people, related to the process of ageing. This is shown in the views and actions of ordinary people and by the actions of institutions of society (Bytheway and Johnson 1990).

Reflection points

● **Using the above definition, what evidence of ageism have you observed in everyday life?**

Thompson (2006) describes a model that identifies discrimination as occurring at three interlinking levels of society: personal, cultural and structural (Figure 2.1):

● *Personal*: ageism is seen at the personal level when individuals use patronising language or avoid contact with older people. It is also evident when older people are not involved in decisions about their care.
● *Cultural*: older people may be depicted in negative terms in all parts of the media. Cruel humour in cartoons and jokes reinforces stereotypes of older people as sick, dependent, childlike, mentally slow and confused.
● *Structural*: ageism at the structural level is demonstrated in institutional policies and practices that perpetuate stereotypes of older people. Services for older people may have lower priority and less flexibility than those for younger people.

Ageism can affect the ways in which older people feel about themselves, resulting in low self-esteem and self-efficacy and low expectations of many aspects of life, including health and social services.

Age discrimination is the most common form of discrimination in Britain. In 2005, 29% of adults of all ages reported experiencing age discrimination, while 24% reported gender discrimination and 19% racism. Age discrimination can be compounded by other forms of discrimination such as in terms of gender, age and ethnicity (Ray et al. 2006). To be older,

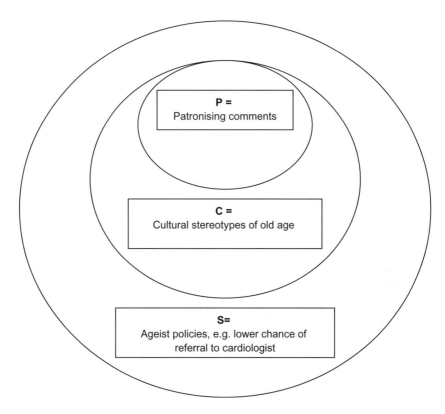

Figure 2.1 Thompson's PCS (personal, cultural and structural) model applied to ageism.

female and a member of an ethnic minority group may attract multiple discrimination: ageism, sexism and racism.

Anti-discrimination law exists to provide protection against racism, sexism and disablism, but there is no equivalent for ageism other than the Employment Equality (Age) Regulations 2006. Under the regulations, there is still a default age of retirement at 65 years, although workers can ask to stay at work after this age. In 2007, the government consulted on a proposed Single Equality Bill that could include age discrimination in the provision of services (including health and social care) and in the provision of goods and facilities (e.g. loans and insurance). The intention is to achieve equal treatment for older people, without sacrificing those concessions which already exist to improve the welfare of older people, such as free bus travel and prescriptions for those over 60 and free television licences for people over 75 (Department for Communities and Local Government 2007).

Ageism in health and social care

Ageism reinforces stereotypical views of older people as lacking competence and being in need of protection (Bytheway 1995). Some, but not all, older people may be seen as 'vulnerable' at various times in their lives. In advanced age, this may be due to physical frailty, lack of resources and their relatively powerless position in society. Services for older people frequently involve risk assessments in order to determine eligibility for services and level of service provision. However, limited availability of resources may result in only those deemed 'high risk' receiving services.

Risk is usually defined in terms of probability of a potential outcome, but services focused on older people may interpret risk as danger to health or well-being. Being categorised as 'at risk' may confer a label on an individual that takes precedence over all other aspects of that person and result in restriction of individual choice (Phillips et al. 2006). In this way, services may reduce independence, and poor services may even create risks for older people. It is important that older people are supported in exercising informed choice about risk-taking in pursuit of maximising their independence (Commission for Social Care Inspection [CSCI] 2006a).

There is evidence that age has been and continues to be a criterion in allocating health resources. The *National Service Framework* (NSF) *for Older People* (DH 2001a) acknowledged that ageism had been experienced by some older people in some areas of healthcare, for example palliative care, trauma care and denial of cardiopulmonary resuscitation.

The UK inquiry into mental health and well-being in later life (Age Concern and Mental Health Foundation 2006) highlighted high levels of unmet mental health needs and few older people receiving services that might help them such as housing, health and social care. The inquiry identified age discrimination in mental health services, such as age barriers to accessing services, poor resourcing of specialist services for older people and failure to address the needs of people growing older with severe mental health problems. Two-thirds of older people with depression never discuss their problems with their GP, and of those who do discuss it, only half are diagnosed and treated. The inquiry concluded that the perception that mental health problems are an inevitable part of ageing needs to be challenged and attention paid to reducing isolation and preventing depression. Age discrimination in mental health services was acknowledged in *Better Health in Old Age* (DH 2004), as was the need for services to be available on the basis of need not age. *Securing Better Mental Health for Older Adults* (DH 2005a) estimated that 40% of older adults attending GP surgeries had mental health problems, as did 50% in general hospitals and 60% in care homes. A Programme Board for older adult mental health services was set up in 2005 to address these issues.

A further example of ageism is illustrated in Harries et al.'s (2007) study of angina in older people. Their research found that 46% of GPs and care of the elderly doctors and 48% of cardiologists treated patients over 65 years differently from younger patients regardless of the coexistence of other disease. Examples given included older patients less likely to be prescribed statins, referred to a cardiologist, given angiography and being offered revascularisation. They were, however, more likely to have their prescriptions changed and be given a follow-up appointment. Interviews with doctors showed that some viewed age as a contraindication to treatment.

Anti-discriminatory practice

Reflection points

- **Think about the care that you provide to older people. How can you ensure that you do not discriminate on the basis of age?**

Hughes (1995) discusses anti-ageist practice and articulates a set of values that should underpin principles and practice. Each older individual is a person of equal value and importance to any other, one who has rights based in citizenship as does any other member of society. Their achievement of a valued stage in life is to be celebrated. Hughes sees these values translating into anti-ageist practice through a set of principles including the promotion of empowerment of older people so that they can have control over their lives and autonomy, leading to self-worth. There should be meaningful involvement and participation in decisions, and choice should be promoted. Older people should be integrated into mainstream life and given every opportunity to live as others, with the same quality of life as other people. The challenge to professionals involved in the care of older people is to translate these principles into practice, in negotiation with older people and their carers.

Thompson (2006) discusses anti-ageist practice for social workers, and this also has relevance for healthcare professionals. He sees the avoidance of ageist assumptions, especially in the assessment of older people, as fundamental. Older people should not be required to adjust to their circumstances, but professionals should seek to empower them rather than making them dependent, acting as advocates and seeking appropriate resources. The use of appropriate language is important, avoiding terms such as 'the elderly' and avoiding infantile terms and endearments.

A holistic approach, promotion of dignity, enhancement of self-esteem and involvement in decision-making should characterise all interactions with older people. Specific guidance for anti-ageist practice in health and social care is provided by the DH in documents such as the *NSF for Older People* (2001a) and campaigns such as Dignity in Care outlined in the *New Ambition for Old Age – Next Steps in Implementing the National Service Framework for Older People* (2006b).

Reflection points

- Think about the life experiences of older people within your family and friendship networks in respect of paid work, voluntary work, income, social life and involvement in the local community.

Employment

Participation in paid work is important for income, security and participation in society, and so has consequences for physical and mental health. In 2004, 12 million people over 50 years were economically inactive. Some, having acquired sufficient financial means, made a positive choice to take early retirement, while others were obliged to cease work due to ill-health or redundancy. Employment in this age group declined substantially in the late 1970s to mid 1990s, but there is now an increase among both men and women, largely in the 50–65 years age group. Older people who have formal qualifications are more likely to be in work than those without qualifications, as are those in higher socio-economic groups. Those who are married or cohabiting are also more likely to be in employment. Self-employment and part-time working are common for older workers (Whiting 2005). Financial necessity caused by the need to pay for basic requirements such as a mortgage, or insufficient pension entitlement, may cause older people in lower socio-economic groups to continue to work (Irving et al. 2005).

Incomes vary over the life course, being lowest in the youngest age group, 16–19 years, rising in early middle age and declining in older age. At all ages, men's income is greater than that of women. Women are more likely to be employed in low-paid work and to encounter obstacles to promotion (Equal Opportunities Commission 2005). Considerable variations can be seen in the incomes of people who have retired from work, with the newly retired receiving more income than those who have been long retired. Just over one-half of average pensioner gross income is made up of benefits, including state pension and Pensioner Credit (Office for

National Statistics 2007). The minimum income for healthy living for those over 65 years without significant disability and living independently is 50% greater than the state pension. It is also appreciably greater than the means-tested Pension Credit guarantee, designed to provide a minimum level of income.

Inadequate income could be a barrier to healthy living for older people in England (Morris et al. 2007). However, most pensioners have some private income in addition to the state pension, for example occupational pensions, with some income from investments and earnings, but few have private pensions (Office for National Statistics 2007). Differences are apparent between gender, with 53% of single female pensioners receiving an occupational or personal pension in addition to a state pension, whereas for men this figure is 66% and for couples 83%. Pensioner incomes have grown faster than average earnings in the last 10 years. However, the Office for National Statistics points out that changes in average income are affected not only by changes experienced by individual pensioners, but also by the impact of newly retired people joining the pensioner group, who have greater entitlement to occupational and private pensions.

People on low incomes often economise, in order to protect small savings and avoid debt, by cutting back on expenditure on clothing and food. This may involve buying cheaper food and using cheaper supermarkets. Cutting back on bills might mean reducing the number of rooms heated or hours of heating (Dominy and Kempson 2006). Such economies may have implications for health.

Poverty in old age is determined by previous experience of employment, income and ability to save and invest. Once older people move into poverty, there is little they can do to improve it. Women's experience of older age is affected by their economic position. Some women have not accrued state pension rights from paid work or been able to afford private pension contributions. This may reflect time spent in caring for family and disjointed participation in paid employment. Women from ethnic minorities are among the poorest pensioners, many of them having no experience of formal employment (Policy Research Institute on Ageing and Ethnicity [PRIAE] 2007). Many women have worked and continue to work in lower-paid jobs. Single women may have had little opportunity to buy their own houses and may lack family support in older age. According to the Economic and Social Research Council, a third of all 1960s Baby Boomers do not contribute to an occupational or private pension, a fifth have no housing wealth, a fifth will be childless and one-tenth will not have married or formed a permanent union (Womack 2005).

Experience of employment is also important for incomes of ethnic minority elders. There are considerable differences between and within groups in terms of occupation. There is a polarisation of Asian

Indians and Pakistani people between professional and managerial occupations and routine occupations. Black Caribbean individuals are clustered in routine and semi-routine occupations (Moriarty and Butt 2004). This has consequences for income and the ability to make provision for older age through occupational or private pensions. In research with older people from selected ethnic minority groups, PRIAE (2005) found that state retirement pensions and social benefits were the main sources of income. Both men and women in minority ethnic groups are less likely to have private pensions than the rest of the population, and this is most marked for those of Pakistani and Bangladeshi origin (Arber and Ginn 2001). Chinese and Vietnamese elders are more likely to experience poverty than African Caribbeans or South Asians (PRIAE 2005).

This discussion provides a brief insight into the differing economic experience of minority ethnic groups. Although 9% of white and 10% of Indian elders are in the richest 20% of the population, many older people experience the cumulative effect of lack of material resources over a lifetime, which may contribute to social exclusion.

Older people may experience social exclusion when they lack some factors that contribute to quality of life (see Figure 2.2). People who have been excluded in adult life may be exposed to worse exclusion in older age, and others may experience social exclusion following bereavement or retirement (Social Exclusion Unit 2006). Those most likely to be affected are women, people living alone, divorced, separated or widowed, those in poor health, those with lower educational levels and those living in a deprived area (Burholdt and Windle 2006). Older people living in socioeconomically deprived areas are more likely to experience cognitive impairment and functional impairment, regardless of their own socioeconomic status (Basta et al. 2008). Those who experience poverty and live in a deprived area may function poorly in terms of self-care, home management and social interaction (Breeze et al. 2005).

Policy as a response to needs of older people

This section starts with a brief explanation of what policy is, prior to discussing relevant agendas and the implications for older people's health and well-being. Policies are said to be 'living things' (Blakemore 1998: 1–2) as they can be concerned with what happens at the coalface of nursing, as well as what happens at strategic level. Policies propose to improve the quality of life of the population, but they can appear unpalatable and controlling (Blakemore 1998). This has some resonance for nurses who are struggling to grapple with changes imposed on them through the implementation of new policies that are attempting to improve the patient experience. Health policy is specifically concerned with directives from the government of the day that respond to the changing health needs of the population, such as those for heart disease, stroke and disability. Government has set individual targets to reduce the incidence of such diseases within a certain time frame (DH 2006b).

Current policy is attempting to address the care of the ageing population within the context of the demographic changes discussed in earlier sections of this chapter. It is becoming more evident that services previously providing health and social care provision for individuals over 60 years are now reducing their age criteria to 50 years and over. It could be suggested that this change reflects the needs of a younger age group who experience statistically more long-term and acute illness.

Changing settings for care

During the last two decades, policy has changed locations where care is provided. As discussed in Chapter 1, large institutions for people with chronic mental illness or learning disabilities, who may or may not be old, have been replaced by smaller community homes. There is also an increasing number of acutely ill older people being cared for in the community. More nurses of all disciplines are now working with older people within the community, either at home, within care homes or within a clinic setting (Denny and Earle 2005). Contemporary care is provided within communities through education, advice and support that require multiprofessional teams. For example, care for older people may require the expertise of generic and specialist nurses, physiotherapists, occupational therapists, voluntary agency workers, doctors, social workers and public health workers. One of the drivers of current policy directives is to improve interdisciplinary and cross-sector working to strengthen links between all health and social care sectors.

There are now fewer hospital beds in the UK, and consequently the majority of older people in society will be cared for in and by the community. They are often not seen as having a medical need and are likely to be discharged from hospital with complex care management needs, requiring a multiprofessional team approach within the community. This not only adds to the pressures of a limited care service provision in the community from both statutory and independent health and social care sectors, but also portrays older people as a burden on a society. This often results in family and friends providing informal care with limited support from the health and social care sectors. A more detailed discussion of this is provided later in the chapter.

Box 2.3 Key themes from policy

1. Choices in care
2. Personalised care
3. Equal access to treatment, services and resources
4. To be treated with dignity and respect

Policy themes

Following the historical perspective discussed in Chapter 1, this section explores policy themes from the year 2000. It is against this demographic and contextual backdrop that *The NHS Plan* (DH 2000a) set out a 10-year plan to reform and improve the patient experience, and it could be suggested that the agendas of most policies released since that time stem from the key principles contained within that document. The policy agendas selected for discussion here demonstrate the impact on both the organisation of services, and on health and social care professionals working with older people in all settings. It is discussed here through the key themes drawn from the policies related directly or indirectly to older people (Box 2.3). It is hoped that this will aid your interpretation of both policy implementation and changes that you experience in practice.

Theme 1: Choice in care

Providing choice about how, when and where older people access their care is a recurring theme through most current policies. Relevant policy documents have been selected here for discussion about these specific agendas.

Choosing Health: Making Healthy Choices Easier (DH 2005c) was released following wide public consultation with individuals, organisations and communities to gain their views on improving health. This policy emphasises three key issues: informed choice, personalised care and working together.

To enable individuals to make their own decisions about choices that impact on their health, better information, support and services to encourage and sustain health improvements are needed. This is seen as especially important for those with mental illness, those with physical disability and those living in poverty, and although not age specific, it is easy to see how these issues are important for older people, through choices about health, access and individual budgets. New initiatives have been established to encourage the public to access health information through their local pharmacies, NHS Direct and Care Direct in addition to their GP.

Choice in care is important to all older people, and as such it is important to discuss what is termed a mixed economy of care. This concept describes the provision of care through different services provided by statutory (National Health Service [NHS] or local authority) and independent services (private, voluntary or charitable organisations). Currently, service provision crosses all these sectors of care. Social care is described as personal care, and healthcare as nursing; however, the boundaries are often unclear and confusing. Social care is mostly means-tested (dependent on income or wealth), resulting in many older people having to pay for their personal care in all settings. Nursing care, however, is free at source. Older people often find this concept difficult to accept when they were promised free care from birth to the grave at the inception of the NHS in 1948.

Reflection points

- **Think of an example of where you have seen older people offered choice in their care. How was it offered? Were there any constraints? Did you feel it was a real choice for this older person or just the best option?**

Theme 2: Personalised care

This involves tailoring services to enable individuals to make choices that suit their individual lives. Personalised care is the right of every individual but is particularly important for people experiencing dementia. Older people with dementia is discussed in more detail in Chapter 6, but in this context personalised care is seen as person-centred care to improve quality of life for individual older people. Person-centred care can be seen from both a negative and a positive stance – as a platform to aid the development of relationship in nursing practice, but also challenging in terms of new ways of working and time constraints (Dewing 2004). Individualised care demands that nurses act as facilitators to ensure that the individual older people retain their sense of identity and autonomy in the provision of their care (Dewing 2004). Hence they become valued as an individual and not seen as an anonymous entity within an homogenous group.

Personalised care for communities can also be seen through a variety of strategies that demand flexibility of service provision that is convenient and easily accessible at local level. The report *A Sure Start for Later Life* sets out to reshape services by bringing them together within communities (Social Exclusion Unit 2006). Sure Start was originally designed for children and parenting, particularly for families experiencing deprivation to enable equal access to services. However, it was realised that this way of working could be beneficial to other age groups in society, and it is currently being piloted in a few areas across England to improve services for older people (Social Exclusion Unit 2006). A Sure Start approach to care for this group of people involves older people themselves being involved in the planning, design and delivery of this community service, which is supported and coordinated by professionals. The principles of this approach involve a flexible service that meets the diverse needs of individuals and provides a single point of access for all services in order to bring together a variety of services that could enhance older people's quality of life.

An example of this approach is in a town in Shropshire where a community centre adjacent to the shopping centre provides a variety of services for older people and is managed by local people. A reception area is run by older people, and there is a café that serves as a drop-in facility and meeting place. A day centre provides care for older people who have recently been discharged from hospital but are not receiving personal social services, for example for bathing. There is also a children's nursery and IT and exercise classes on site that provide services for the whole community. This is an example of a purpose-built service involving older people from its inception, to ensure that relevant individualised services are provided on site. In addition to access to care and treatment, there is also a great emphasis on prevention of ill-health, specifically for older people in their community (Social Exclusion Unit 2006). This example highlights the importance of inclusivity for equal access of services for older people.

Theme 3: Equal access to treatment, services and resources

Although there have been some improvements in access to care, there remain elements of discrimination against older people accessing services. AGE – The European Older People's Platform (2004) looked at older people's experiences of discrimination in access to services across Europe. For example, they found that age limits were set for access to some screening procedures. Age limits to free breast-screening, for example, were present in most member countries (65 years in the UK). They also found that clinical trials for cancers often excluded older people even though a third of cancers occur in the over 75s. The *NSF for Older People* (DH 2001a) demands that health and social care services must be based on clinical need and not on age. This document addresses the structure of services and as such sets out national standards of care for older people in all settings. When considering health and need for care, the *NSF for Older People* recognises three broad groups (Box 2.4).

Box 2.4 Age groups covered by the *NSF for Older People* (Department of Health 2001a)

- *Those entering old age*, who have completed their careers in paid employment and child-rearing, who may be 50–65 years old and still active and independent
- *Those in a transitional phase* between a healthy active life and frailty, who may be in their 70s or 80s. These individuals need care designed to identify problems at an early stage, as well as an effective response that will prevent long-term dependency
- *Frail older people* who are vulnerable as a consequence of physical or mental health problems, probably in late old age

There is still much work to do to achieve the standards within the *NSF for Older People* to eliminate age discrimination. In *A New Ambition for Old Age – Next Steps in Implementing the National Service Framework for Older People* (DH 2006b), the review of progress showed that although many more older people were able to access services and treatments, and overt age discrimination was uncommon, there were 'still deep rooted negative attitudes and behaviours towards older people' (p. 2). *Living Well in Later Life* (Healthcare Commission 2006) identifies that ageism can still be seen in examples such as: patronising and thoughtless treatment by staff; poor standards of care on general wards; poorly managed discharges; repeated movement from one ward to another for non-clinical reasons, and meals taken away before older people can eat them. It is suggested by the BBC (2006b) that the NHS remains ageist because society remains ageist.

The document *Our Health, Our Care, Our Say* (DH 2006a) is concerned with a government agenda of more effective health and social services. An extensive consultation paper was undertaken to gain public views. This policy also reflects similar agendas of choice, personalised care and services closer to people's homes. However, it places great emphasis on shifting care and facilities away from hospitals to community settings such as new community hospitals. This concentrates on improving the quality of services in localities and making them more responsive to the needs of the local population. As with other policies, partnership working is seen as imperative to improve choices and health, but here there is an emphasis on shared responsibilities between social services and health providers. A policy to provide individual budgets and direct payments for care has emerged from this paper, providing opportunities for individuals to choose and pay for their care.

Theme 4: To be treated with dignity and respect

'Dignity in care' is defined by Levenson (2007) as 'the kind of care, in any setting, which supports and promotes, and does not undermine, a person's self-respect regardless of any difference' (p. 9). Issues of dignity and respect have been prominent in many of the policy documents since the *NSF for Older People* (DH 2001a). *The New Ambition for Old Age* initiative (DH 2006b) is seen as the next steps in implementing the *NSF for Older People*. Practice-based leaders are now accountable for ensuring that older people are treated with respect for their dignity in maintaining high standards of care, particularly in care for mental health problems (Age Concern 2007) and at end of life (NHS 2006).

Public consultation with older people has given them the opportunity to speak out about the lack of dignity and respect given to older people within health and social care. As a result, a group of dignity guardians have been set up to improve the regulation of social care (*Time to Care*, CSCI 2006b). BBC Radio 2 commissioned a survey of 1000 people aged 16 and over in 2006. More than half of all the respondents believed that there was a great deal of neglect and mistreatment of older people in Britain, a percentage that rose to 60% among female respondents (BBC 2006a). According to those polled, the majority of neglect and mistreatment occurred in care homes (53%) and hospitals (48%). One in 10 cited examples of physical abuse. Cases of older people being left unfed and humiliated were also highlighted (BBC 2006a).

Policy is trying to address and prevent the abuse and mistreatment of older people through two documents. The Protection of Vulnerable Adults (POVA) scheme was explained within the Care Standards Act 2000 (Office of Public Sector Information 2000). A practical guide to the POVA Scheme (DH 2006c) document provides details of how care agencies and businesses are required to request checks against the POVA list as part of the Criminal Records Bureau disclosure process (p. 7). The POVA scheme aims to prevent the employment of inappropriate caring personnel to not only registered adult care providers, but also care homes and domiciliary care organisations who register with the Commission for Social Care Inspection (or Care Standards Inspectorate in Wales) (DH 2006c: 8).

The POVA Scheme reinforces the *No Secrets* (DH 2000b) guidance document that sets out processes to follow should there be a suspicion of abuse or maltreatment. All local authorities jointly with their local NHS trusts across England and Wales were directed to develop and publish their own document for their care staff.

As will be discussed more fully in Chapter 3, the Mental Capacity Act 2005 (Office of Public Sector Information 2005) also defines a new criminal offence of ill-treatment or wilful neglect of a person over 16 years old lacking capacity. A crime of this magnitude in any care setting could result in a term of up to 5 years' imprisonment. These strategies have been put in place to prevent the abuse and mistreatment of older people on discharge from hospital, at home and within care homes.

Health and social care provision

This section explores care provision within various settings. It demonstrates how NHS reforms are promoting new ways of working and associated new roles. Evidence is also provided of older people's experiences of care.

Current government agendas aim to enhance care and promote independence for older people in a variety of settings. This includes enabling older people to remain in their own homes, reducing hospital stays and preventing the 'revolving door' whereby older people are readmitted to hospital within 48 hours of discharge. Opportunities for new roles have emerged to implement these agendas. The introduction of the community matron and the new type of worker such as the assistant practitioner are examples of these new roles introduced to meet these current agendas for older people (DH 2004, 2005b).

Intermediate care schemes for older people have been introduced at home and within some care homes to assist in rehabilitation, enabling older people to return to their own homes after an incident affecting their health or well-being. Intermediate care was set out in the *Supporting Implementation – Intermediate Care* document (DH 2002). It aimed to ensure that a range of integrated services were in place to ensure rapid recovery from illness, prevent hospital admissions and promote independent well-being for individuals in their own homes.

Care at home

There is much evidence that older people wish to remain and receive care in their own home, and healthcare services have sought to achieve this where feasible through community nursing and community matron roles (DH 2005b). Deciding the best options for older people and their families is often stressful, and there are some examples of where although a care home may be the most appropriate place, it has been excluded from discussions to avoid spending the 'children's inheritance'. The reality of care can, however, still remain with the family, who may feel a responsibility to care (because of filial responsibilities).

Macdonald (2003) found that health and social care service provision at home could be variable as it was dependent on professionals or the individual being aware of local services available to them. Some older people were reluctant to call in formal care, preferring to call on friends and relatives. This could result from a concern about becoming a nuisance or losing their independence (Themessl-Huber et al 2007). Home care was valued, but older people thought that there was only limited time to meet their needs before they left to go to somewhere else (Themessl-Huber et al 2007).

Research by PRIAE (2005) into the use of health and social care by selected groups of black and minority ethnic elders showed that satisfaction with health services was high overall. Chinese/Vietnamese individuals used GPs, district nurses, day care and home care considerably less frequently than other groups. This might have been due to a greater reliance on Chinese medicine or concern about using UK services due to a lack of awareness of the free services available to all.

All groups wanted to be treated with respect, avoid delays and have information in their own language. African Caribbean elders made most use of day care services – 80% – compared with 44% of South Asians. Frequent users had better health, less pain and more self-esteem, and satisfaction with services was high. Over-75s were less satisfied than the younger group. The PRIAE (2005) report emphasised the need to address language barriers. It recommended that social care should have clear charging policies, but that many ethnic group members would be too poor to be required to pay. The poor use of services by Chinese and Vietnamese elders needs further research, and stronger policies on equity need to be developed by all providers (PRIAE 2005). Within the same research, black and minority ethnic organisations identified reasons for unmet needs among black and minority ethnic elders including language problems, lack of information, inadequate services and staff lacking multicultural/intercultural competence. Black and minority ethnic elders were seen to lack understanding of the complex service structure, which is often difficult enough for people who have lived all their lives in the UK to understand.

The increasing number of older people from ethnic minority groups points to the need to discuss and plan with them services that will meet the diverse needs of ethnic elders. There is a need to overcome the stereotype that black and minority ethnic communities 'look after their own'. Families within these communities face their own pressures in everyday life – such as work, childcare and poverty – that may affect their ability to provide informal care.

Care in extra-care housing, residential and nursing homes

Care for older people on discharge from hospital is increasingly being provided at home, with only 4.5% (Office for National Statistics 2005) entering a care home. Institutional settings include residential homes, nursing homes (termed as care homes) and extra-care housing. Extra-care housing is currently becoming a favoured choice of housing provision for older people by both local councils and older people themselves. It offers purpose-built housing for older people in either a flat or bungalow, or in part of a retirement village complex, where care can be provided in situ. It can provide a sense of independence and the potential for older people to retain their identity (CSCI 2006c).

Residential homes provide individual or shared rooms with communal living facilities to meet personal needs. Nursing provision can also be made, from district nurses to community matrons as required. The new type of worker role is becoming commonplace in residential care homes, where healthcare assistants are gaining skills to undertake work previously provided by district nurses. An example of this can be seen in some local authority residential homes where the new type of worker can utilise skills of phlebotomy, spirometry and complex wound management (Kessler and Bach 2007). This shift in care provides continuity of care for residents and links to local primary care trust staff that provide the training.

Reflection points

- How do older people and their relatives decide on where they receive care? Where do they get information on care?
- Discuss with colleagues how they perceive institutional care. Where did they acquire this perception, and has it changed over time?

As a result of government agendas to reduce hospital stays and the closure of long-term hospital beds, care homes are rapidly becoming nurse-led units for residents with complex high-dependency health and social care needs. As autonomous workers, nursing staff need to be highly skilled to meet these needs, in addition to having the leadership and management skills required in the independent sector.

Decisions in accessing long-term care in either residential or care homes have been problematic for older people and their carers. Understanding where money is allocated in care homes has eluded many older people and professionals alike. In the CSCI study *A Fair Contract with*

Older People (CSCI 2007), evidence was collated from older people in care homes and their families and carers. The study revealed that there were some examples of where appropriate information was accessible about care provision to aid decision-making on entering a care home. However, there were some instances when older people and their families were unable to gain sufficient information or support in making a decision about entering a care home. Payments for care in care homes were not always overt and clear, which was not helpful at a time of stress and urgency to find an appropriate care setting for an older person (CSCI 2007). This is often compounded by examples of where older people have had to remain in hospital because of lack of an appropriate place to stay and have therefore been labelled as 'bed-blockers'. The impact of this on older people adds to the burden they may feel on both the healthcare system and their family. The recommendations from this study are set to ensure that older people and their families have access to independent advice and support through brokerage services on a one-to-one basis (CSCI 2007).

Resident's experiences of living in a care home are included in *My Home Life* (Owen and National Care Homes Research and Development Forum 2006), a report on quality of life in care homes. Testimonies showed that residents valued independence and sought to achieve this within the structure and routines of their Care home. Although some people chose to reside in a care home, others had sought to avoid being a burden on relatives or felt they had been forced to do so. One resident, originally from the Caribbean, having made the decision to live in a care home, found it hard to adapt at first, but found that it gave her more friends than she had had when living in her own home. She felt she had made the right choice despite the fact that she could no longer have the food she loved – rice and peas or pork with gravy – although this had been available when she was in hospital. She was eagerly awaiting a prosthesis for her leg stump so that she could be more independent of the care staff for her daily care needs.

Residents praised staff, who were seen to be caring, but some found few other residents with whom they could converse. Days were reported as being mundane, although many homes attempted to provide activities and entertainment. Having everything done for them in the care home meant that there was a lot of expertise and skills among the residents that was now wasted. Lack of adequate 'pocket money' for those receiving benefits meant that they had difficulty in phoning family (who used mobile phones) or giving presents at Christmas.

Residents wanted to be able to communicate their wishes about their environment and needs in relation to entertainment with staff. They also wanted the opportunity to talk about death and express grief when someone in their family or in the care home died. Mention was also made of the use of 'patronising' language by young staff members.

Box 2.5 Four key indicators for National Health Service-funded nursing care (Department of Health 2007b, 2007c)

1. The nature of the condition
2. The complexity of symptoms
3. The intensity of needs
4. The unpredictability of the condition.

Choices about where older people are cared for are dependent on need and who pays for care. Elders are often concerned that they should have sufficient funds to pay for their funeral and would prefer to go without to ensure that they retain this sum of money. As a result, many older people are still outraged by the cost of care and concerned about spending their money in this way as it may be taking money away from what the family sees as their inheritance. Some older people may feel that they should die rather than see all the money disappear into their care (Vincent 1999). Payment for long-term care is very complex, and no attempt has been made here to provide the actual cost of health and social care. In brief, nursing care is free to all in any setting (DH 2007b, 2007c); however, there are strict criteria to access this funding. A standard assessment of needs determines whether an individual meets the criteria through four key indicators (Box 2.5).

NHS-funded care is provided by a registered nurse either at home or in a care home. Nursing care provision includes a detailed examination and assessment of identified health needs, the monitoring and planning of individual care plans, support for self-medication and medication as required (DH 2007b, 2007c). For older people who are not assessed as needing nursing care from a registered nurse, there is still a system in which individuals are means-tested by the local authority to decide who pays for care and how much. Means-tested systems have always been unpopular for older people, who may not wish to disclose their financial situation and therefore prefer to pay the full rate of payment for personal care services at home. Even for those who feel able to discuss their financial circumstances, some or all of the payment may still remain within their responsibility. The current debate as to what is deemed a nursing need and what is a social or personal need may indeed continue, especially around the needs of people with dementia, who are not seen as having a nursing need solely because of their condition. The setting in which older people find themselves is often dependent on resources available rather than their specific choice. It is also dependent on their ability to fund their long-term care or rely on relatives and social services to fund their care services.

Results of a study by Boyle (2004) found that choice in services could be dependent on whether you lived at home or in a residential or nursing home. Boyle found that older people who lived alone at home received more choice in care, which included filial care. However, choice could also be restrained by dependency on care staff or family in terms of time, willingness and ability to care. So choice was not always about what care was to be received, but also about when and where. This study also revealed that older people living in institutional care appeared to have more choice in activities than those living at home.

Realities of service provision

The realities of service provision can often differ from a theoretical perspective. The previous section examined the role of policy, its development and implementation. Here, consideration is given to who actually does the caring within this policy agenda and the experiences of individuals living with care provision.

People's experience of care is somehow dependent on: whether they live alone; family structure; how their health is medicalised; where they live; and their gender. In terms of medicalisation, older people may find their house overwhelmed by medical equipment such as commodes and hospital beds, making normal family life more difficult. Independence for older people is important. However, Shah (2002) puts an argument forward to promote more medicalisation of older people. He stresses that offering more medicine could reduce the morbidity and mortality of older people. Therefore, reducing medicine on the grounds of age could place more cost on the health system, in addition to reducing quality of life for older people.

Older people and rurality is also an issue for discussion globally. Alston (2002) highlights how people living in rural areas have less choice about their care services, and how distance is a problem for access to service provision, both formal and informal.

Filial responsibilities

There was a plethora of literature expounding on filial (informal family) caring and responsibilities in the late 20th century (Ungerson 1987), but it tended to focus on the negative experiences of carers. This seems unhelpful in exposing some benefits for both the older person and their family carer (Donorfio and Sheehan 2001). In their study, Donorfio and Sheehan found that caring for ageing parents was influenced by individual cultural values and caring expectations, although the responsibility still seems to lie with the children of the family, particularly daughters and daughters-in-law. This has been reinforced in many other studies (Coward and Dwyer 1990; Spitze and Logan 1991). It also suggests that daughters change their relationships with their mothers to set the caring limitations for them. Benefits of caring for older parents relate to a sense of purpose (Walker et al. 1995), the development of closer relationships and an opportunity to develop a renewed relationship (Walker et al. 1990). Mutual feelings of well-being and appreciation were expressed in a study of relationships between ageing mothers and daughters (Donorfio and Sheehan 2001).

There is also evidence that older people themselves may not wish to see their family carer becoming burnt out and stressed, and may feel that they are burdensome and no longer wish to live. Similarly, it must be acknowledged that not all families have good relationships with their ageing dependant, and where this exists, the older person may no longer want to live in this dependency relationship (Vincent 1999).

Current patterns of family life in the UK are changing in ways that may affect the provision of care for older people. Care by families often means care by women, but men participate in caring for older relatives too, particularly spouses (Fear 2001). Being married is important here for older people today as it provides not only social support, but also a resource for practical caring responsibilities. This may of course change for future generations where different types of family form exist that may complicate who takes on the caring responsibility. A study by Coleman and Ganong (2002) demonstrated that, even with ageing divorced parents, the adult children felt some form of responsibility for care.

Older people may be divorced, and some will have remarried or entered new partnerships, but others living alone may experience restricted sources of informal assistance and support. Potential carers may also divorce, and remarriage or new partnerships may affect perceptions of caring responsibilities for step-parents. Divorce may also affect older people's financial situations in retirement and old age, and many women are now involved in paid work outside the home; this may restrict the time available for informal caring.

Older people as carers and users

Currently, more than 1 million people over 65 years receive publicly funded social services in England (Wanless 2006). However, the story is more complex than this as a third of these older people themselves are also providing care for significant others (Baggott 2004). In reality, older people not only receive informal care, but are also involved in providing unpaid care. There are 1.2 million men and 1.6 million women over 50 years old providing care for others (Office for National Statistics 2007). Older people are said to provide care for spouses and family members. In terms of longevity, older people after retirement age are providing more and more care for their aged parents. This is in addition to increasingly caring for grandchildren while sons and daughters are in employed work (Polett et al. 1991). Even though this work is well documented, older people's status in UK society remains devalued. Many older people contribute voluntary hours as part of the mixed economy of care (Hoad 2002) through caring for family members of all ages (Polett et al. 1991).

Reflection points

- Do you know of older people who provide care for another? Discuss with them or your colleagues how caring may affect health and well-being? How may these effects be addressed?

As the largest users of NHS services, older people are sometimes seen as a burden to society. As suggested by Taylor and Field (2003), older people's use of health services dramatically increases over 75 years of age. They also report that although older people do not necessarily experience difficulties in accessing primary healthcare services, this may not equate with a quality or satisfactory provision of appropriate services. Older people sometimes feel that both health and medical practitioners do not listen to their needs (Berney et al. 2000). Older people with long-term conditions have gained considerable knowledge about their diseases. This is acknowledged by government, and self-care is promoted through *The Expert Patient* (DH 2001b).

Conclusion

The provision of appropriate support services is essential to ensure a good quality of life for increasing numbers of older people in the community. Constraints on financial resources are set to continue, and the challenge will be to implement policy agendas within limited NHS resources.

Currently, Scotland and Wales are funding institutional care, but England has to date resisted pressures to follow suit. This issue will remain on the political agenda for discussion over time, but there remains the challenge of where sufficient funds can be found for service provision for older people in all settings.

Government agendas are seeking to promote the inclusion of older people, choice in care, equal access, personalised services, and dignity and respect. This includes models of working designed to encourage self-care (DH 2005b). It could be suggested that government agendas have increased expectations of and demands for service provision; hence, there may be implications for families in providing increased support and care.

There has been constant change in service provision, and this seems set to continue into the future. Challenges can be anticipated in designing services that enhance care and address discrimination for older people, who are now the largest group in our society. There are also challenges for existing staff and those in new roles to meet the ever-changing complex needs of older people in a variety of settings.

References

Acheson, D. (1998) *Independent Inquiry into Inequalities in Health.* Available from http://www.archive.official-documents.co.uk/document/doh/ih/contents.htm

AGE – the European Older People's Platform (2004) *Age Barriers, Older People's Experiences of Discrimination in Access to Goods, Facilities, and Services.* Available from http://www.ageconcern.org.uk/AgeConcern/Documents/AGE_doc_goods_and_services_2_Dec_2004.pdf

Age Concern (2007) *Improving Services and Support for Older people with Mental Health Problems.* Available from www.ageconcern.org.uk

Age Concern and the Mental Health Foundation (2006) *Promoting Mental Health and Well-being in Later Life: A First Report of the UK Inquiry into Mental Health and Well-being in Later Life.* Available from http://www.mhilli.org/index.aspx?page=stage2promotion.htm

Alston, M. (2002) Social capital in rural Australia. *Rural Society* 12(3): 93–104.

Arber, S. and Ginn, J. (2001) Pension prospects of minority ethnic groups: inequalities by gender and ethnicity. *British Journal of Sociology* 52(3): 519–39.

Baggott, R. (2004). *Health and Health Care in Britain*, 3rd edn. Basingstoke: Palgrave.

Basta, N.E., Matthews, F.E., Chatfield, M.D. and Brayne, C. (2008) Community-level socio-economic status and cognitive and functional impairment in the older population. *European Journal of Public Health* 18(1): 48–54.

BBC (2006a) *Older people survey.* Available from http://www.bbc.co.uk/pressoffice/pressreleases/stories/2006/06_june/05/elders.shtml

BBC (2006b) *Battle Lines Drawn over Discrimination Laws*. Available from http://news.bbc.co.uk/1/hi/business/6039744.stm

Berney, L., Blane, D., Davey-Smith, G. and Holland, P. (2000) Life course influences on health in early old age. In H. Graham (ed.) (2000) *Understanding Inequalities in Health*. Buckingham: Open University Press.

Blakemore, K. (1998) *Social Policy: An Introduction*. Buckingham: Open University Press.

Bytheway, B. (1995) *Ageism*. Buckingham: Open University Press.

Bytheway, B. and Johnson, J. (1990) On defining ageism. *Critical Social Policy* 10(29): 27–9.

Boyle, G. (2004) Facilitating choice for older people in long-term care. *Health and Social Care in the Community* 12(3): 212–20.

Breeze, E., Jones, D.A., Wilkinson, P. et al. (2005) Area deprivation, social class, and quality of life among people aged 75 years and over in Britain. *International Journal of Epidemiology* 34(2): 276–83.

Burholdt, V. and Windle, G. (2006) *The Material Resources and Wellbeing of Older People*. York: Joseph Rowntree Foundation.

Chandola, T., Ferrie, J., Sacker, A. and Marmot, M. (2007) Social inequalities in self reported health in early old age: follow up of prospective cohort study. *British Medical Journal* 334: 990–6.

Coleman, M. and Ganong, L. (2002) Resilience and families. *Family Relations* 51(2): 101–2.

Commission for Social Care Inspection (2006a) *Making Choices, Taking Risks*. Available from http://www.carestandards.org.uk/PDF/making_choices_taking_risks_companion_paper.pdf

Commission for Social Care Inspection (2006b) *Time to Care*. Available from http://www.csci.org.uk/PDF/time_care_full.pdf

Commission for Social Care Inspection (2006c) *The Extra Care Housing Toolkit*. Available from http://www.integratedcarenetwork.gov.uk/_library/Resources/Housing/Support_materials/Toolkit/ECH_Toolkit_Website_Version_Final.pdf

Commission for Social Care Inspection (2007) *A Fair Contract with Older People: A Special Study of People's Experiences when Finding a Care Home*. Available from http://www.csci.org.uk/PDF/fair_contract.pdf

Coward, R. and Dwyer, J. (1990) The association of gender sibling network composition and patterns of parent care by adult children. *Research on Ageing* 12(2): 158–81.

Denny, E. and Earle, S. (2006) *Sociology for Nurses*. Cambridge: Polity Press.

Department for Communities and Local Government (2006) Table 1.3 in *Housing in England 2004/05*. Available from http://www.communities.gov.uk/documents/housing/pdf/153388.pdf

Department for Communities and Local Government (2007) *Discrimination Law Review: A Framework for Fairness: Proposals for a Single Equality Bill for Great Britain – A Consultation Paper*. Available http://www.communities.gov.uk/publications/communities/frameworkforfairnessconsultation

Department of Health (2000a) *The NHS Plan: A Plan for Investment, a Plan for Reform*. Available from http://www.dh.gov.uk/en/Publicationsandstatistics/Publications/PublicationsPolicyandGuidance/DH_4002960

Department of Health (2000b) *No Secrets: Guidance on Developing and Implementing Multi-agency Policies and Procedures to Protect Vulnerable Adults from* Abuse. Available from http://www.dh.gov.uk/en/Publicationsandstatistics/Publications/PublicationsPolicyAndGuidance/DH_4008486

Department of Health (2001a) *National Service Framework for Older People.* Available from http://www.dh.gov.uk/en/Publicationsandstatistics/Publications/PublicationsPolicyAndGuidance/DH_4003066

Department of Health (2001b) *The Expert Patient: A New Approach to Chronic Disease Management for the 21st Century.* Available from http://www.dh.gov.uk/en/Publicationsandstatistics/Publications/PublicationsPolicyandGuidance/DH_4006801

Department of Health (2002) *The National Service Framework for Older People: Supporting Implementation – Intermediate Care: Moving Forward.* Available from http://www.dh.gov.uk/en/Publicationsandstatistics/Publications/PublicationsPolicyAndGuidance/DH_4006996

Department of Health (2004) *Better Health in Old Age.* Available from http://www.bjhc.co.uk/telecare/docs/Better%20health%20in%20old%20age%20(DoH).pdf

Department of Health (2005a) *Securing Better Mental Health for Older Adults.* Available from http://www.dh.gov.uk/en/Publicationsandstatistics/Publications/PublicationsPolicyAndGuidance/DH_4114989

Department of Health (2005b) *Supporting People with Long Term Conditions: An NHS and Social Care Model to Support Local Innovation and Integration.* Available from http://www.dh.gov.uk/en/Publicationsandstatistics/Publications/PublicationsPolicyAndGuidance/DH_4100252

Department of Health (2005c) *Choosing Health: Making Healthy Choices Easier.* Available from http://www.dh.gov.uk/en/Publicationsandstatistics/Publications/PublicationsPolicyAndGuidance/DH_4094550

Department of Health (2006a) *Our Health, Our Care, Our Say: A New Direction for Community Services.* Available from http://www.dh.gov.uk/en/Publicationsandstatistics/Publications/PublicationsPolicyAndGuidance/DH_4127453

Department of Health (2006b) *A New Ambition for Old Age: Next Steps in Implementing the National Service Framework for Older People.* Available from http://www.dh.gov.uk/en/Publicationsandstatistics/Publications/PublicationsPolicyAndGuidance/DH_4133941

Department of Health (2006c) *Protection of Vulnerable Adults Scheme in England and Wales for Adult Placement Schemes, Domiciliary Care Agencies and Care Homes: A Practical Guide.* Available from http://www.dh.gov.uk/en/Publicationsandstatistics/Publications/PublicationsPolicyAndGuidance/DH_4134725

Department of Health (2007a) *Health Survey for England 2005. The Health of Older People: Summary of the Findings.* Available from http://www.ic.nhs.uk/webfiles/publications/hseolder/HSESummary.pdf

Department of Health (2007b) *National Framework for NHS Continuing Health-care and NHS-funded Nursing Care.* Available from http://www.dh.gov.uk/en/Publicationsandstatistics/Publications/PublicationsPolicyAndGuidance/DH_076288

Department of Health (2007c) *NHS Continuing Healthcare and NHS-funded Nursing Care Public Information Booklet.* Available from http://www.telford. gov.uk/NR/rdonlyres/C1B8ED48–8405–46AF-8186–9A2B771AB494/0/ DOHCHCInfoLeaflet.pdf

Dewing, J. (2004) Concerns relating to the application of frameworks to promote person-centredness in nursing with older people. *Journal of Clinical Nursing* 13(3a): 39–44.

Dominy, N. and Kempson, E. (2006) *Understanding Older People's Experiences of Poverty and Material Deprivation.* Department of Work and Pensions Research Report No. 363. Available from http://www.dwp.gov.uk/asd/asd5/ rports2005–2006/rrep363.pdf

Donorfio, L. and Sheehan, N. (2001) Relationship dynamics between aging mothers and caregiving daughters: filial expectations and responsibilities. *Journal of Adult Development* 1(1): 39–49.

Economic and Social Research Council (2007) *Adding Quality to Quantity: Older People's Views on their Quality of Life and its Enhancement.* Available from http://www.esrcsocietytoday.ac.uk/ESRCInfoCentre/Plain_English_Summaries/ LLH/index140.aspx?ComponentId=9577&SourcePageId=11772

Equal Opportunities Commission (2005) *Free to Choose: Tackling Gender Barriers to Better Jobs. England Final Report.* Available from http://83.137.212.42/ sitearchive/eoc/PDF/occseg_finalrep_england.pdf?page=17446

Fear, T. (2001) Male or female carers: differences and similarities. *Journal of Dementia Care* 8(4): 28–30.

Giddens, A. (2006) *Sociology.* Cambridge: Polity Press.

Harries, C., Forrest, D., Harvey, N., McClelland, A. and Bowling, A. (2007) Which doctors are influenced by a patient's age? A multi-method study of angina treatment in general practice, cardiology and gerontology. *Quality and Safety in Health Care* 16: 23–27.

Healthcare Commission (2006) *Living Well in Later Life: A Review of Progress Against the National Service Framework for Older People.* Available from http://www.healthcarecommission.org.uk/_db/_documents/Living_well_in_ later_life_-_full_report.pdf

Hoad, P. (2002) Drawing the line: the boundaries of volunteering in the community care of older people. *Health and Social Care in the Community* 10(4): 239–46.

Huber, J. and Skidmore, P. (2003) *The New Old. Why Baby Boomers Won't Be Pensioned Off.* London: Demos.

Hughes, B. (1995) *Older People and Community Care: Critical Theory and Practice.* Buckingham: Open University Press.

Irving, P., Steels, J. and Hall, N. (2005) *Factors Affecting the Labour Market Participation of Older Workers: Qualitative Research.* Department of Work and Pensions Report No. 281. Available from http://www.dwp.gov.uk/asd/ asd5/rports2005–2006/rrep281.pdf

Jagger, C. (2000) Compression or expansion of morbidity – what does the future hold? *Age and Ageing* 29: 93–4.

Kessler, I. and Bach, S. (2007) *The Skills for Care New Types of Worker Programme: Stage 1 Evaluation Report.* Available from http://www.topssengland. net/files/NToW%20st1%20eval%20report%20web%20edn.pdf

Levenson, R. (2007) *The Challenge of Dignity in Care, Upholding the rights of the Individual, A report for Help the Aged.* Available from http://policy. helptheaged.org.uk/NR/rdonlyres/7368AC05-4CCD-4165-873D-4282083BA783/0/upholdingrights101007.pdf .

Macdonald, T. (2003) *The Social Significance of Health Promotion.* London: Routledge.

Mold, F., Fitzpatrick, J.M. and Roberts, J.D. (2005) Minority ethnic elders in care homes: a review of the literature. *Age and Ageing* 34(2): 107–13.

Moriarty, J. and Butt, J. (2004) Inequalities in quality of life among older people from different ethnic groups. *Ageing and Society* 24: 729–53.

Morris, J.N., Wilkinson, P., Dangour, A.D., Deeming, C. and Fletcher, A. (2007) Defining a minimum income for healthy living (MIHL): older age, England. *International Journal of Epidemiology* 36(6): 1300–7.

National Health Service (2006) *End of Life Programme.* Available from http://www.endoflifecareforadults.nhs.uk/eolc/

Nazroo, J., Bajekal, M., Blane, D., Grewal, I. and Lewis, J. (2003) *Ethnic Inequalities in Quality of Life at Older Ages: Subjective and Objective Components.* Available from http://www.esrcsocietytoday.ac.uk/ESRCInfoCentre/ Plain_English_Summaries/social_stability_exclusion/index147.aspx? ComponentId=9589&SourcePageId=11733

Office for National Statistics (2005) *Focus on Older People.* Available from http://www.statistics.gov.uk/focuson/olderpeople/

Office for National Statistics (2007) *Social Trends* No. 37. Available from http://www.statistics.gov.uk/

Office of Public Sector Information (2000) Care Standards Act 2000. Available from http://www.opsi.gov.uk/acts/acts2000/en/ukpgaen_20000014_en_1

Office of Public Sector Information (2005) Mental Capacity Act 2005. Available from http://www.opsi.gov.uk/ACTS/acts2005/ukpga_20050009_en_1

Owen, T. and National Care Homes Research and Development Forum (2006) *My Home Life, Quality of Life in Care Homes.* London: Help the Aged.

Pensions Commission (2005) *Pensions: Challenges and Choices.* Available from http://www.dwp.gov.uk/mediacentre/pressreleases/2005/feb/belfast-pn1702. pdf

Phillips, J., Ray, M. and Marshall, M. (2006) *Social Work with Older People,* 4th edn. Basingstoke: Palgrave Macmillan.

Policy Research Institute on Ageing and Ethnicity (2005) *Black and Minority Ethnic Elders in the UK Health and Social Care.* Available from http://www.priae.org/projects/bmeelderssecretariat.htm

Policy Research Institute on Ageing and Ethnicity (2007) *Policy Response to the Healthcare Commission's Gender Equality Scheme.* Available from http://www. priae.org/publications.htm

Polett, P., Anderson, I. and O'Connor, D. (1991) For better or for worse: the experience of caring for an elderly dementing spouse. *Ageing and Society* 11: 443–69.

Ray, S., Sharp, E. and Abrams, D. (2006) *Ageism: A Benchmark of Public Attitudes in Britain.* Available from http://www.ageconcern.org.uk/AgeConcern/ Documents/Ageism_Report.pdf

Roberts, Y. (2004) *Fifty is the New Thirty . . . So Drop the immer frame Jokes.* Available from http://www.guardian.co.uk/uk/2004/may/23/britishidentity. focus

Shah, E. (2002) The medicalisation of old age. *British Medical Journal* 324: 861–3.

Social Exclusion Unit (2006) *Sure Start to Later Life: Ending Inequalities for Older People.* Available from http://www.communities.gov.uk/documents/corporate/pdf/913275.pdf

Spitze, G. and Logan, J. (1991) Sons, daughters and intergenerational social support. *Journal of Marriage and the Family* 46: 901–7.

Taylor, S. and Field, D. (2003) *Sociology of Health and Health Care,* 3rd edn. Oxford: Blackwell.

Themessl-Huber, M., Hubbard, G. and Munro, P. (2007) Frail older people's experiences and use of health and social care services. *Journal of Nursing Management* 15(2): 222–9.

Thompson, N. (2006) *Anti Discriminatory Practice.* Basingstoke: Palgrave Macmillan.

Townsend, P. and Davidson, N. (1982) *Inequalities in Health.* Harmondsworth: Penguin.

Ungerson, C. (1987) *Policy is Personal: Sex, Gender and Informal Care.* London: Tavistock Publications.

Victor, C.R. (2005) *The Social Context of Ageing.* Oxford: Routledge.

Vincent, J. (1999) *Rethinking Ageing: Politics, Power and Old Age.* Buckingham: Open University Press.

Walker, A., Pratt, C. and Eddy, L. (1995) Informal caregiving to aging family members: a critical review. *Family Relations* 44(4): 402–11.

Walker, A., Shin, H. and Bird, D. (1990) Perceptions of relationship changes and care giver satisfaction. *Family Relations* 39(2): 147–52.

Wanless, D. (2006) *Securing Good Care for Older People: Taking a Long Term View.* London: King's Fund.

Whiting, E. (2005) The labour market participation of older people. *Labour Market Trends* 112(6): 285–96.

Womack, S. (2005) Women are the old-age losers. *The Edge* 20: 28–30.

Chapter 3

Ethical tensions for the older person and carers

Lesley Moore

Introduction

For the past decade, there have been various White Papers, research documents and debates about end of life issues affecting the older person, and examples of how older people are often excluded and abused in society (House of Commons Health Committee 2004; Smith 2005; O'Keefe et al. 2007). The ethical issues and tensions that arise are often rooted in values and beliefs that can lead to conflicts and dilemmas for the older person, carers and professional staff. Many older people will come into contact with healthcare professionals through health promotion initiatives, or as a result of being treated for acute or long-term conditions. They may be dwelling within their own homes, in a carer's home or in a residential or care home. Wherever they are dwelling, it is important that professionals understand their values and beliefs and respect their rights and culture.

This chapter will explore the influencing factors that affect: priorities of values and beliefs; the paradigm shifts that are still evolving; the power dimensions in healthcare relationships; the impact of new laws, such as the Mental Capacity Act (Ministry of Justice 2005), and the contemporary debate of end of life care and decision-making.

Paradigm shifts in health and social care

Tensions are a part of everyday life, as change is a part of working life. However, as ethical understanding evolves due to the embedding of a rights culture, it is important for healthcare professionals to reflect on and learn of the impacts of paradigm shifts of change, so that they can move with, and influence, change in the future. Journeying and learning through change can raise many cognitive, emotional and ethical tensions that can be likened to the analogy of change eras, known as paradigms of transition, where there are changes from one way of thinking and doing to another over a period of time (Kuhn 1970).

A learner, whether qualified or unqualified for a professional role, undertaking specific education and training could experience the tide of change in both education and practice. In practising skills of inquiry and reflection during such paradigm shifts, it is important for the learner to gain awareness of ethical knowledge (especially of self; Noddings 1984), the changing paradigms within healthcare, and boundaries within communities of practice (Wenger et al. 2002). As paradigm shifts develop new values, so dilemmas and tensions and a different priority of ethical principles and new knowledge may emerge. Some of the tensions arise as new roles evolve and learners, while developing their skills, start to cross boundaries, sometimes witnessing 'tribalistic' behaviour (Moore 2007). Tensions can also arise when boundaries are misinterpreted, and personal and organisational values and beliefs conflict.

Figure 3.1 is a simple Venn diagram of the shifting paradigms in healthcare. Paradigm X reflects the traditional picture of healthcare based

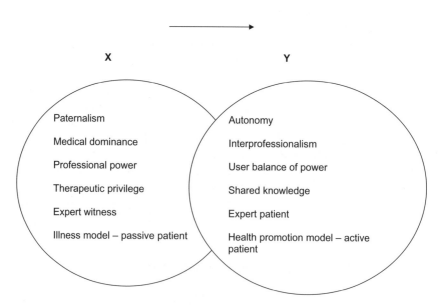

Figure 3.1 Paradigm shifts in health care.

on an illness model and paternalism. The latter is a situation in which doctors viewed the patient as having a disease or ailment that needed to be treated and they knew what was in the patient's best interest (Campbell et al. 1999; Beauchamp and Childress 2001). Often the ethical justification was that the principle of beneficence was a priority (Beauchamp and Childress 2001). So, in the doctor–patient relationship, it was doctors who dominated and claimed powerful control based on their scientific medical knowledge. This science gave them the therapeutic privilege, based on specialist knowledge, to make decisions in isolation and deny patients the right to make informed decisions (Veatch 1981), rendering them passive recepients of care. A situation that Illich (1987) referred to as disabling but one that raises many tensions in the workplace, which, sadly, as we have seen in the Bristol Inquiry (Kennedy 2001) and the Shipman Inquiry (Smith 2005), result in negative health outcomes and closed rather than open practices. The era of traditional paternalism is still alive in some National Health Services (NHS) sectors but, according to Levy (2008), it is 'strictly time-limited', as changes are effected (p. 50)

There could be another tension evolving with radical thinking if another form of paternalism is not considered. As can be seen in Figure 3.1, the two paradigms overlap. Seedhouse (1988) suggests that it may cause more problems if the paradigms go in different directions. There is a need for the recognition that a different kind of paternalism may be required during the span of patient–doctor relationship. For example, an older man with chronic obstructive pulmonary disease experiences an exacerbation of his condition following a cold spell of weather. Struggling to breathe, he seeks help from his GP. In reading the situation, knowing that answering many questions will tire the patient, the GP may make a decision in the patient's best interest to admit him to hospital or change his medication. At this stage, the patient is vulnerable, the exacerbation disabling him in making decisions for himself, so he accepts the doctor's actions based on 'moral trustworthiness' (Campbell et al. 1999, p. 19). It could be argued that, by involving the doctor at this time, he has given implied consent to paternalistic care and decision-making at a time when he may not have been able to reason. This differs from traditional paternalistic behaviour, in which consent was not sought, information was not explained and actions were not explained to the patient.

In Figure 3.1, paradigm Y reflects the shift towards a health model in which the ethos is one of autonomy, and where the patient and healthcare professionals learn to work together towards a goal of better health. The patient is respected as an intelligent person and receives appropriate knowledge to make informed choices on how to manage their health, and to have a say in the redesign of care services. This is particularly important and empowering for older people with long-term conditions (Department of Health [DH], 2005). A partnership model for integrated care needs a special relationship where there is compassion and empathy, and recognition of diversity and support for equality and inclusiveness, especially in decision-making (Healy 2001; DH 2000a, 2005; Youngson 2008). The diversity should be inclusive of people with learning, physical and mental disabilities. There is a vision of professional groups working with patient groups in which the professionals reflect integrated team characteristics (Miller et al 1999) such as being able to:

- work interprofessionally according to a shared vision
- support power-sharing
- work within and across role boundaries that are flexible according to patient requirements.

This vision is one that NHS reforms are working towards. Such characteristics suggest that team players would have the ability to reason with confidence and competence, and to respect one another's opinions (Stephenson and Weil 1992). The quote from Miller et al. (1999) may reflect the virtues of an interdisciplinary team, but there is another form of power-sharing to consider. This is a shift in which the user of healthcare gains more power in the decision-making process and is also recognised as a 'a greater moral authority' as the recipient of care (Youngson 2008: 6). It is this shift that may cause more moral tensions as the philosophy of *The Expert Patients Programme* (DH 2006b) and consumer choice (DH 2006a) embeds, and some staff do not shift to working within paradigm Y.

According to Seedhouse (1988), the slogan for the autonomy paradigm Y should be 'work for health is a moral endeavour' (p. 17). It is this paradigm which Seedhouse stated 'has not yet crystallized' (p. 10), but it is fair to point out that, in recent years, the momentum towards this paradigm has gathered more speed as the Modernisation Agenda for the NHS has been implemented. This has led to the need for many transformations in learning to learn in the workplace. One of those transitions is the inclusion of patients and carers in group work that is focused on change. Kohner (1996) suggests that group work could focus on ethical issues that require wider debate and could include both patients and carers. However, she does recognise that some professionals may not find this desirable, but, as she argues, it is essential and requires sensitive handling and organisation. Significant learning can be gained by health and social care staff from actively listening to the opinions of the service user, particularly in understanding the myriad influencing factors that may affect their decisions, morality, values and beliefs.

Table 3.1 Factors Influencing moral reasoning and behaviour

Personal values	Cultural values and beliefs
Finance	Age
Experience of life	Religion
Politics	Travel
Law	Professional codes
Schooling/education	Media
Prejudices	Illness

Factors influencing moral reasoning and behaviour

As Table 3.1 indicates, there are many societal influencing factors that can contribute to both moral reasoning and behaviour. Those indicated in Table 3.1 are but a few that have gained attention in recent White Papers and research concerning the vulnerability of older people, especially those with mental health problems such as dementia (House of Commons Health Committee 2004; La Fontaine et al. 2007; O'Keefe et al; 2007).

From this list, some of the factors have been developed further. The following reflection may help you to consider more factors.

Reflection points

- Take some time to reflect on your experiences and identify other influencing factors that you could add to this list. Alternatively, draw a spider diagram with 'influencing factors' in the body. Each factor could contribute to an extra leg.
- Then consider the possible impacts of these factors on the service user–health professional relationship.

Values and beliefs

Within a multicultural society such as the UK, the understanding of human rights and respect of the person is very complex, especially if the older person's values and beliefs conflict with those of the people giving care.

A value can be interpreted as a quality that is regarded highly by an individual and is worthy of respect. With other values, a person will develop a system or set of beliefs that have been influenced by many factors. Throughout life, a person will prioritise the system of values and beliefs according to their experience of life (Rokeach 1969). It is these values that influence a person's choices and direction in life. Fry (1994) identifies that values may be non-moral or moral in nature. An example of non-moral value may be cleanliness or efficiency, whereas a moral value could include, for example, honesty and respect. Both moral and non-moral values may be reflected in personal, cultural and professional values (Burnard and Chapman 1988).

A conflict arises when a person's set of values and beliefs clashes with those of others. For example, a nurse may value cleanliness (non-moral) and expect all residents living in a care home to bathe daily. An older man may, however, value his freedom (moral) to choose whether or not to bathe daily. The nurse is now faced with a dilemma in that there is more than one action she can take. Her decision should be made according to what the older man believes is in his best interest, and in so doing the nurse will need to weigh up any risks, harms and intrusion into his rights. A registered nurse is advised by her Code of Practice, which stipulates that she must justify any acts or omissions (Nursing and Midwifery Council [NMC] 2008).

Similarly, a new GP examines an older Asian man in his home. His professional judgement, based on what he believes is in the patient's best interest, is that the patient should receive palliative care in a local community hospital or hospice to manage his pain relief. This may be a Western cultural value that could conflict with an Asian cultural value of caring for family in the community. The GP may also not have considered alternative actions whereby a community palliative care team could manage the pain relief in the home, or in some cases the patient might prefer to meditate at home. The latter may be a cultural value and ritual in managing pain that may not be valued by Western medicine.

Another example is where the second and third generations of minority ethnic groups may in time come to value the benefits of Western medicine. A conflict within the family who are caring for an older relative may arise when medicine such as Chinese remedies may be favoured by the elder in preference to modern medicine. The elder may not have learnt the host language of the country he or she is living in. A tension may arise for community practitioners when family carers attempt to speak on behalf of the older person. In such situations, it is easy for family carers to express their own values instead of those of the older person. Behind closed doors, the tension within families may lead to coercion and abuse. This type of behaviour is not new, for as Hek (1998) identified, the abuse often recognized by district nurses could be 'physical, psychological, social or financial' (p. 131). Such behaviour may be accepted within the family as a norm, making it more difficult for the district nurses to read the situation and decide what to do.

As can be seen by these examples, ethical tensions can arise when different values conflict. What is important as a first step towards understanding ethical tensions and decision-making for developing professionals is time to reflect and explore their own values concerning the older person (Fry 1994), and to consider ethical theories that may influence decision-making, as well as the myriad social factors influencing moral reasoning.

Reflection points

- Reflect on your own personal, cultural and professional values, especially those regarded as a priority. Identify which are non-moral and which are moral.

Significant ethical theories

At the policy and professional levels of healthcare in the UK lie three significant ethical theories that have had an impact on decision-making, namely deontology, utilitarianism and rights. The first two theories have dominated decision-making in healthcare for many years, whereas the rights theories and the Human Rights Act (Office of Public Sector Information 1998) are just starting to make an impact.

The word deontology arises from the Greek word, *deon*, which means a duty. The most notable deontologist was Immanuel Kant. At the centre of his ethics was 'the exercise of freedom and good will in an action', which was moral if enacted from a sense of duty (Thompson 2005: 91). This sense of duty has underpinned many healthcare codes of practice (Seedhouse 1988; Campbell et al. 1999). The duty within a community would be that all persons must be respected as persons and not treated as a means to an end (Curtin and Flaherty 1982). So it would be wrong for a healthcare practitioner to befriend an older person (who is a patient) and coerce them to make a will identifying the practitioner as the main beneficiary. This would be an example of using the patient, as a means, to gain a personal wealth, an end.

The deontological theory is based on intentions of goodwill, but does not consider how some people may act in given situations, or take account of any consequences that may arise from some actions. This nonconsequential approach is a disadvantage of the theory and the codes of practice that it underpins. It does not consider how conflicts and dilemmas can be addressed (Curtin and Flaherty 1982; Seedhouse 1988; Campbell et al. 1999; Thompson 2005). Scenario 3.1, adapted from Campbell et al. (1999), highlights a conflict between rights and duties.

Scenario 3.1: Conflict between rights and duties

Agnes, an elderly lady with severe dementia, in fact almost vegetative, is in a rest home. She suffers a fractured neck of femur, a stroke and pneumonia . . . she is dying, a priest visits her to administer the final absolution. He requests her nasogastric tube be removed while he gives her water, and this is done. Just as he is finishing, the nurse returns and reinserts the tube because it is time for Agnes' afternoon feed and it is the nurse's duty not to hasten her death. Ten minutes later, Agnes dies.

The nurse has followed what she perceives as her duty and has not considered any possible consequences.

Reflection points

- Reflect upon Scenario 3.1 and make a note of what you may consider to be any consequences of these actions for Agnes and her family.

Agnes has a right to a dignified death, which for her and the family may mean her right to religious last rites. The nurse may have a duty to care not to hasten her death, but by reinserting the tube she has not considered the possible consequences for Agnes, such as suffering and discomfort. If her relatives were present, they might have interpreted this final act or duty of the nurse as an intrusion of Agnes' right for a peaceful death. A question arises of why the nurse had to act at the time that she did. It may be that the nurse was driven by task orientation to fulfil her duty. This situation is a good example of where the patient's rights may come into conflict with the duty of the nurse.

As Curtin amd Flaherty (1982) identified, the master utilitarian Jeremy Bentham maintained that 'people should act to maximize pleasure and minimize pain' (p. 51). According to utilitarian theory, laid down by Bentham, what makes an act right or wrong depends on the principle of utility (Curtin and Flaherty 1982; Thompson 2005). Bentham, a British social reformer of the 19th century, was concerned for the social good of any moral actions, which had to be useful and benefit the majority of society. In Agnes' case, the fact that she died so shortly after the reinsertion of the tube to feed her could be considered by supporters of utilitarianism as unnecessary.

It is the consideration of consequences of an act that underpins the early utilitarian philosophy of Bentham. Another underlying principle is 'the greatest happiness for the greatest number' (Campbell et al. 1999: 5). A later utilitarian, John Stuart Mill, recognised a place for rules in assessing acts as right or wrong. He believed, for example, that the rule 'one should tell the truth is a general means of securing the greatest happiness for the greatest number' (Thompson 2005: 81). This particular rule could be broken in 'exceptional circumstances', such as withholding 'bad news from someone who is dangerously ill, for fear of causing him or her harm' (Thompson 2005: 81). The principles of beneficence – for the benefit of – and nonmaleficence – to do no harm – are two more that are valued by utilitarians.

Decision-makers and economists at the policy level of primary care trusts may use utilitarian methods to ensure that monies are spent to ease the suffering of the greatest number of patients within their locality. For example, there may be two young, married men needing heart transplants, and at least 100 men and women between the ages of 65 and 75 years requiring hip replacements (Seedhouse 1988). A formula, known as quality-adjusted life years has been used for many years. This is based on the cost, risk and benefits to society (Williams 1985; Maynard 1987). Campbell et al. (1999) suggest that a man of 75 years could lose out to a man of 45 years regarding certain medical treatments. Today, this ageist approach could be challenged by the Human Rights Act (Office of Public Sector Information 1998).

However, in the larger number example, there are more complex perspectives to consider. The cost of the heart transplants and their sustaining medicines and monitoring mechanisms could provide a life expectancy of 10–20 years for the two men. Some may argue that there are other social benefits to consider in that these men may have responsibilities for young families, as opposed to the pensioners who have brought up their families and had a 'fair innings' (Campbell et al. 1999: 139). In considering the amount of money required for hip replacements for the older age group, the cost of the surgery could be less than that for the two men requiring a heart transplant. The potentiality for older people to recover and still contribute to society could be a far greater saving than maintaining the life of two young men with expensive drugs. Populations are living longer, and following retirement many older people are caring for grandchildren or supporting charity organisations. The critics of the utilitarian method of quality-adjusted life years in managing the health purse claim that it is unethical on the basis that an individual's right to healthcare is being denied, and the method could be used to discriminate against certain groups such as older people, (Harris 1987; Rawls 1989).

The rights movement in the UK has been quite contentious. A right is a 'justified claim that individuals and groups can make upon others or upon society' (Beauchamp and Childress 2001: 50). A claim to a right implies that another person or party is obliged to satisfy that right. Over 200 years ago, Thomas Paine (1987) believed that, according to man, 'His natural rights are the foundation of all his civil rights'. Even then, he was trying to sow the seed that the natural rights of food, shelter, welfare and healthcare should be secured by law. However, his critics at the time, such as Bentham, believed that natural rights were 'nonsense on stilts' (Waldron 1987: 166). Bentham's four charges against rights (Waldron, 1987: 166) were that:

1. '. . . human rights are unduly abstract in their formulation – that they abstract too much from locality, history and the detailed circumstances of human life;
2. . . . theories of rights are too rationalistic – they exaggerate what can be achieved by reason in political philosophy;
3. . . . these theories are too individualistic in their approach to social life; and
4. . . . needs to be carefully distinguished from the third, that the idea of rights introduces an unjustified element of egoism into moral argument.'

These utilitarian criticisms were made at a time in history when poor houses existed for many older people who had worked for many years for a pittance and had no means to support their retirement. Thomas Paine's values were shunned by British politics, but he was later influential in the design of the American Bill of Rights.

However, the criticisms of rights are still used today by politicians when considering health and social care systems. The most common one is the fourth charge, which has often led to a destruction of family relationships when a member has 'become preoccupied with their own individual entitlements' (Waldron 1987: 188). In such situations, it can be those who are more vulnerable, such as older people, who could become more isolated and, when in need of care, have no option but to live in a care home.

The rights movement in the 20th century was fuelled further by three dominant theories:

- the social contract theory of justice (Rawls 1973)
- the political theory of distributed justice (Nozick 1974)
- the work of Dworkin (1977), who supported a legal approach to uphold a Bill of Rights.

These are dominant in that they have influenced the thinking of UK political parties.

Rawls (1973) interprets justice as fairness, the 'primary subject' of which is the 'basic structure of society' (p. 7). Rawls (1973) believed that moral members of society would strive to maximise their primary goods, which he categorised as natural and social primary goods. The natural goods, which he regarded as the basic structure of society, included, health, vigour, intelligence and imagination. The social primary goods included rights, liberties, powers, opportunities, income and wealth. His first principle prioritises liberty and the social goods, and the second principle recognises social and economic inequalities that, within society, should be arranged so that they are both:

a) to the greatest benefit of the least advantaged, consistent with the just savings principle, and
b) attached to offices and positions open to all under conditions of fair equality and opportunity. (p. 302)

So this suggests that citizens have to be active in providing for their future. This approach was certainly valued by the Thatcher government of the 1980s. With wealth, citizens would be able to pursue their liberties. However, in the case of older people who have lost capacities such as intelligence and imagination due to cognitive impairment, they would not be in a position to pursue such liberties. Their assets may have been used to support their care if they have been admitted to care homes, but this may render them poor in economic terms. Rawls (1973) does recognise support for poverty through his difference principle, but once again the person would need to be able to give something back to society in the form of work. So Rawls' contract theory does little to support the health and social care of most vulnerable older people.

Nozick (1974) believed that people have a right to food, clothing, shelter and medical care as these are distributable goods. He did not support claims to a natural right of good health and a good life as these are not distributable goods. His theory is based on the following three principles:

1. The principle of (initial) acquisition of holdings
2. The principle of transfer
3. The principle of rectification.

These principles support the right of individuals to acquire possessions and properties without infringing the rights of others. Once in possession of such goods, the owner can decide what to transfer and to whom. This would protect hereditary rights and would challenge any decisions, which has happened recently where savings and homes have been used to pay for the social care of a spouse, leaving the remaining spouse in a poorer situation. Nozick (1974) would consider this to be a violation of rights, and this is where the third principle would come into play. This would be a right for the situation to be rectified. What this theory does not cater for are those who cannot help themselves or provide monies to care for them. It leaves the vulnerable ones in society to be at the mercy of communities who decide whether or not to care for them. It would be permissible within this theory for communities to make such judgements.

It is perhaps Dworkin's (1977) theory of rights that 'defends individual rights' (p. 271) and brings us closer to a Bill of Rights or Act that supports the growth of a fair and just society. Fundamental to a fair society and antidiscrimination is the 'right to equal respect and concern' (p. 82). However, on their own, such principles are somewhat abstract and would lack argumentative power. Dworkin felt that the right to liberty within the UK, the right to choose, was under threat by utilitarian-led governments. Once protected by moral laws, he maintained that the individual rights such as equal respect and concern could act as 'political trumps' over utilitarian decisions. Although the UK was a member of the European Convention of Human Rights, Dworkin (1990) felt that by a specific Bill of Rights drawn up by British judges there could be 'a more generous interpretation, using the rich and special traditions of the British common law to develop out of the Convention a particularly British view of the fundamental rights of citizens in a democratic society' (p. 22). If there were such a Bill or Act, the arguments would be appropriate for public services such as the NHS.

It was to be another 8 years before the Human Rights Act 1998 in the UK received Royal Assent and came into force in October 2000. Table 3.2 lists various Articles within the Act. It is important to note that the right to health is 'enshrined' in the Universal Declaration of Human Rights (Hancock, 2000: xii), and with the Human Rights Act it was forecast that the relationship between patient, secondary and primary healthcare teams would change considerably (Wilkinson and Caulfield 2000).

Issues such as the NHS complaints procedure, the treatment of older people, the closure of care homes and access to information relating to public health issues, identified by the then Association of Community Health Councils for England and Wales, had remained unresolved for many years. Chester (2000) hoped that the Act would help to resolve these. However, it takes time to develop a rights culture in both the NHS and social care workforces and the community. Policy-makers, executive health teams, professionals and stakeholders have a responsibility to monitor and challenge the embedding of the rights culture in society.

There are at least five of the Articles of the Human Rights Act 1998 by which the NHS and its employees could be held to account, particularly in relation to the older person. The five principles relating to the Articles have been identified in *Human Rights in Healthcare – a Framework for*

Table 3.2 Articles of the Human Rights Act 1998

Article	Title
1	Obligation to secure rights and freedoms
2	Right to life
3	Prohibition of torture, or of inhuman or degrading treatment or punishment
4	Prohibition of slavery and forced labour
5	Right to liberty and security
6	Right to a fair trial
7	No punishment without law
8	Right to respect for private and family life
9	Freedom of thought, conscience and religion
10	Freedom of expression
11	Freedom of assembly and association
12	Right to marry
14	Prohibition of discrimination
16	Restrictions on political activity of aliens
17	Prohibition of abuse of rights
18	Limitations on use of restrictions of rights

Table 3.3 Relationship between principles and Articles of the Human Rights Act 1998

Principle	Human Rights Act Article
Dignity	3. Right not to be tortured, or treated in an inhuman or degrading way
Equality	14. Right not to be discriminated against in the enjoyment of other human rights
Respect	8. Right to respect for private and family life
Autonomy	2. Right to life
	8. Right to respect for private and family life
Fairness	6. Right to a fair trial

Local Action (DH 2007a). Table 3.3 shows the relationship between the principle and the appropriate Article.

Although the framework (DH 2007a) includes examples of policy or practice change, these will increase in time as practitioners and users of health and social care begin to explore the rights and new laws that will evolve. The Act itself could change in time with the needs of society. The language of Article 2, for example, emphasises that the law safeguards a right to life, and this does not necessarily rule out a form of euthanasia (Wilkinson and Caulfield, 2000). Civil law does recognise the full autonomy of an adult of sound mind to make decisions about life. So if a patient refuses to take medication that could keep him or her alive, the law will support this decision. Such a decision should be respected, recorded and communicated appropriately by healthcare professionals.

Power versus professional perspectives

Scenario 3.2 describes an incident that could occur in any setting. It is an example of negative power that was fuelled by a nurse's ignorance of legal perspectives that could protect her and the patients' rights, a care manager's ignorance of the law, and the obvious abuse of the resident. In considering accountability, there have been many reports in the last decade that highlight abuse of patients, especially of those with mental health problems such as dementia (Dimond 1997; Smith 2005).

Recently the new NMC Code for Standards, Conduct, Performance and Ethics (2008) identifies that the nurse's first concern is the care of people, 'treating them as individuals and respecting their dignity' (p. 1). The nurse in Scenario 3.2 was following the rules of accountability regarding her concern for the patients' dignity, comfort, cleanliness and risk of infection, and she was able to justify her actions to the care home manager. However, by crossing an unfamiliar care boundary, she had not kept abreast of the standards and means of monitoring to which managers of care homes were subject. This gap in her knowledge made both the patients and herself more vulnerable to abuse.

Scenario 3.2: Abuse of human rights and ethical principles

A newly qualified staff nurse has secured a position on a medical ward. To address her mounting debt, incurred through her course, she has also agreed to undertake one night shift a week in a care home for people with dementia. On the first shift, she identified that the gentlemen on the top floor shared one face flannel. In the morning, she asked the care manager for more flannels for each individual person.

The following week, she found that this request had not been addressed, and that night some men suffered diarrhoea and vomiting. To resolve the situation of a lack of personal flannels, the nurse decided to cut up hand towels. In the morning, she informed the manager of her actions and explained why. The manager's response was to sack her for misappropriation of property, and the threat that she would be reported to her professional body and could be removed from the register. The young nurse was extremely upset and eventually confided in her ward sister. The sister listened to the facts and supported the nurse in contacting the local care homes inspectorate.

Reflection points

- **What were the values that concerned the nurse?**
- **What principles and human rights were abused?**
- **What were the ethical tensions?**
- **Who is accountable for what, and what responsibilities do you think the care home manager, ward sister and nurse have?**

A more positive example of power will evolve when patients receive appropriate information to enable them to determine health outcomes, especially at the end stage of life. Making a decision on which care home to choose is a huge task and major life event for both the older person and their family. Nyberg (1981) forecast that patients would be in more control of information to inform their decision-making – the ultimate power over power – but this was slow to materialise in the 20th century. As healthcare practitioners are advancing their practice, it is timely for them to turn to a more expanded interpretation of power, argued by Chinn (1995), in which it is seen in a more positive light of empowering and enabling individuals to take more responsibility for their decision-making, especially at the end stage of life.

Moore (1999) in a small study, identified that a minority of community and hospital nurses showed a willingness to empower patients in end of life decisions, and some saw an advance statement as giving some credence to the process, but they were still concerned about the legal dimensions of the duty to care. The British Medical Association's (BMA; 1995) *Advance Statements about Medical Treatment* recognised the need for improved communication and the need to debate issues within the team and with significant others, BMA members being advised not to make decisions in isolation. Although this advice was not law at the time, it did demonstrate a shift in thinking towards more multidisciplinary working.

In recent years, new White Papers, agencies and statutory powers have been introduced to raise the patients' voice in the NHS arena. As Levy (2008) has pointed out, there is still a long way to go to achieve this positive power. Scenario 3.3 reflects current problems that some vulnerable people may experience in trying to maintain independence in the community because of an imbalance of powers.

Scenario 3.3: Maintaining independence in the community

A retired husband and wife have recently moved into a village. It has proved difficult for the couple to socialise in the community as the husband has mild dementia. During his lucid moments, he is able to collect the daily newspaper from the shop at the end of the road. However, he does at times wander into homes and cars that have not been locked. Some villagers have escorted him to his bungalow and reunited him with his distraught wife. Others have verbally and physically abused him as they have pulled him from their cars. Recently, he has been found wandering on a major trunk road. Worried villagers have spoken to the police and the wife regarding his vulnerability. The couple do not have children and the wife is becoming quite distressed.

At the outset of his diagnosis his wife and a niece agreed to be made and registered as Lasting Power of Attorneys (LPAs). Previously, her husband was experiencing more lucid moments while taking the drug Donezipil. To the wife's dismay, the GP withdrew the drug following recommendations from the National Institute for Health and Clinical Excellence (2006). The local GP has advised her that her husband needs to be cared for in a nursing home. She is reluctant to accept this and is willing to try other methods such as technology to help her care for her husband.

Reflection points

- **How can a positive power be promoted in this situation?**
- **What are the communication hurdles that need to be addressed?**
- **What agencies are involved in this situation?**

Underpinning the new Mental Health Act (Office of Public Sector Information 2007) are five statutory principles that serve to protect people who lack capacity. According to the *Mental Capacity Act 2005 Code of Practice* (Ministry of Justice 2005), a person's capacity or lack of is defined as 'their capacity to make a particular decision at the time it needs to be made' (p. 19).

The principles will challenge traditional paternalistic decision-making as they were designed to enable patients to participate in decision-making where possible. The onus is on those caring for patients with limited or diminishing cognitive powers to continually assess their capacity to make decisions and to take practicable steps to include them in decision-making processes (Ministry of Justice 2005). It will be important for carers not to assume incapacity on the grounds of unwise decisions made by patients (Ministry of Justice 2005). In situations where the patient does not have the mental capacity to make decisions, the law emphasises the centrality of the patient's rights as indicated in the last two principles:

4. An act done, or decision made, under this Act for or on behalf of a person who lacks capacity must be done, or made, in his best interests.
5. Before the act is done, or the decision is made, regard must be had to whether the purpose for which it is needed can be as effectively achieved in a way that is less restrictive of the patient's rights and freedom of action. (p. 19)

As LPAs, the wife and niece would have been registered with the Office of the Public Guardian and Court of Protection. The latter can appoint a deputy if the wife should die before her husband. The LPA differs from the previous Enduring Power of Attorney (EPA) in that its powers continue after the patient has lost capacity to make decisions. As LPAs, the wife and niece have a responsibility to work jointly to manage personal health and welfare, property and financial affairs for the patient. This is another difference in that the EPA covered only property and financial affairs. Those registered as LPAs have a duty to follow the statutory principles.

As his wife, the woman is in a position to carefully assess his mental capacity, for example to shop for the paper and handle money, or to help with household chores, on a daily basis. It may be that she is aware that he gets confused about shares and income tax inquiries. Complex decisions such as these would be covered by the wife's responsibility under the LPA. It could be argued that the GP may not be in a position to assess the patient's mental capacity on a daily basis, but it would be important for him and other agencies involved, such as social services and the community mental health team to work closely with the wife and niece to monitor any deterioration or developments, and to advise appropriately and according to the statutory principles.

The withdrawal of available therapies for people with progressive dementia appears to reflect medical decision-making in isolation, based on biased randomised controlled trials and monetary concern (Royal College of Nursing [RCN] 2005). A response by the RCN emphasised the need for more qualitative research to establish the impact on the patient's and carer's quality of life. The patient's and carer's voice and experiences could provide positive evidence of the value of medication in promoting a better quality of life and retaining personhood (RCN 2005). In making such responses, the RCN later joined forces with the Alzheimer's Society and the Royal College of Psychiatrists, an example of collaborative working in the interests of people with dementia. The couple in Scenario 3.3 may benefit from more joined-up thinking and working between health and social care, and the use of technology discussed in Chapter 7.

End of life and decision-making

National and international law regarding end of life decision-making has been criticised for being 'inconsistent and sometimes incoherent' (McLean 1996: 262). The issue of advanced directives or living wills has been and is currently a major challenge for healthcare and the law.

In 1996, the United Kingdom Central Council for Nursing, Midwifery and Health Visiting (UKCC) defined advanced directives as 'documents made in advance of a particular condition arising and they show the patient's or client's treatment choices, including the decision not to accept further treatment in certain circumstances' (NMC 2006: 2; UKCC documents are no longer available, the organisation now having been superseded by the NMC.)

Although there was no statute on this issue at the time, common law in Great Britain recognised that there was a legal force and parallels with the laws of consent and trespass to person. So if a practitioner chose to ignore a living will and, without consent, instigated treatments, this would be interpreted by common law as assault and battery. Within some groups of healthcare practitioners, there was a call for a new law to overtly support living wills.

The BMA code of practice regarding Advance Directives (1995) was drawn up in response to a request by the House of Lords Select Committee on Medical Ethics (1994). The code evolved from debates between senior nurses, doctors and lawyers. Table 3.4 indicates the types of advance statement that the working party explored. Types E and F were the ones supported by common law and the professional bodies at the time. A qualitative study of 39 nurses working in acute and primary care trusts found that only nine identified the legal force of type E and F advance statements (Figure 3.2; Moore 1999).

The research tool was a collection of vignettes focused on situations of the older person at the end stage of life. Advance directives and living wills were used interchangeably in the research (Moore 1999). The majority of nurses stated that there was no legal force of living wills; this is perhaps not surprising when 18 identified that they had had no opportunity to explore the legal aspects and only nine had recently discussed such issues with colleagues and patients. Two of these issues were focused on

Table 3.4 Types of advance directives identified by the British Medical Association (1995)

Type	Description
A	Requesting or authorising treatment
B	Stating general values based on the individual's beliefs and aspects of life
C	Stating preferences as to how the person would like to be treated
D	Naming a friend or another person who should be consulted at the time a decision has to be made
E	A clear instruction refusing some or all medical procedures
F	A statement that, rather than refusing any particular treatment, specifies a degree of irreversible deterioration after which no life-sustaining treatment should be given

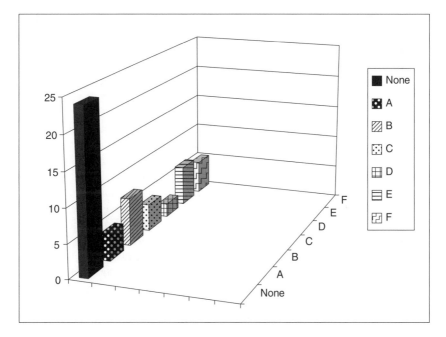

Figure 3.2 Types of living will (A–F; see Table 3.4) believed to have legal force (*n* = 39) (Moore 1999).

recent media coverage. These findings suggest a paucity of knowledge and an indication that the nurses were unable to make the link between the ethical and the legal principles when focusing on an ethical situation. Making links is an important skill that enhances reasoning ability.

Since the launch of the Mental Capacity Act (Ministry of Justice 2005), a type D directive has been added to E and F as supported by law. Another change is that the terminologies of 'advance statements' and 'living wills' have been replaced by 'advance decision.' The previous terminologies were used to reflect written statements prepared by the patient. The new terminology covers both verbal and written decisions. The Mental Health Act 2007 *Draft Revised Code of Practice and Secondary Legislation* (DH 2007b) raises the importance of the family. If the decision is verbal, it will be important for healthcare staff to make an accurate recording, but in both cases the advance decision to refuse medical treatment must be 'valid and applicable to current circumstances' (p. 158). Those patients who are or may be detained under the Mental Health Act 2007 cannot use advance decisions to refuse treatment for their mental disorder.

In the case of advance decisions for patients of sound mind to refuse treatments, healthcare and social care practitioners have a responsibility to establish whether the patient has an advance decision, and the patient too has a responsibility to inform his or her GP of its existence. Where the refusal is for life-sustaining treatment, this has to be explicitly written, witnessed, signed and stored in the patient's file. Some doctors may find that this is against their religious beliefs and ethics, but the code is explicit in that although they can object and not act against their beliefs, they must not 'abandon' the patient but have a duty to pass the patient to another doctor without jeopardising the patient's care.

A contentious issue during the discussions for drafting the BMA code of practice (1995) was 'basic care', and whether or not patients had the right to refuse in advance or instruct others to refuse on their behalf. The working party decided that patients should not be entitled to these rights due to possible unacceptable consequences that could harm the patient and others. However, it was acknowledged that the interpretation of 'basic care' was problematic and needed 'careful consideration', and that professionals should provide what is 'reasonable'. This part of the debate indicated the complexity of the ethicolegal minefield of multidisciplinary practice. The clarity of thought was cloudy at the macro levels of healthcare decision-making in respect of advance statements.

Since then, the *Mental Capacity Act 2005 Code of Practice* (Ministry of Justice 2005) has clarified that artificial nutrition and hydration is medical treatment and can therefore be refused. Basic care is interpreted as the essential care to maintain the comfort of the patient. This includes 'warmth, shelter, actions to keep a person clean and the offer of food and water by mouth' (p. 167). A written advance decision cannot refuse basic care, but at the time of dying a patient cannot be forced to eat and drink as this could be interpreted as assault and battery. The patient still reserves the right to refuse at the time, according to common law. Reference to the *Mental Capacity Act 2005 Code of Practice* and the BMA code (1995) may help health and social care staff to understand some of the diversities and tensions of caring.

The diversities and tensions of caring

As the modernisation of the NHS unfolds, traditional roles and boundaries will need to change. Specialist nurses in cardiac and respiratory care have already moved from secondary care into primary roles as community matrons (Moore 2007). Others, including some community nursing staff, have moved into integrated services and are leading intermediate care initiatives (Wile et al. 2003). Changing contexts and undertaking new roles can lead to many tensions (Hudson and Moore 2006; Moore 2007). The current debate by Levy (2008) on an independent NHS that is driven by public consultation and involvement, if implemented, could cause more ethical tensions for caring. This could be evident in situations where the different types of caring are not acknowledged and respected by some in healthcare teams, and not aligned with what the patients want. Table 3.5 indicates a synthesis of research findings by the Picker Institute (Levy 2008) of the eight domains of the patient's highest priorities. These reflect the need for more joined-up thinking and working of professionals with relevant stakeholders. All of the domains are applicable to caring for the older person in the community, but there are tensions that need to be addressed if the final transition to the end stage of life is to be what the patient wants.

Moore (2000) identified expressed views from Dutch nurses that primary nursing had helped them to develop the skills of empathy and caring, to the extent to which they felt they were close enough to the patient to explore innermost feelings and fears. Such a situation promotes a type of human interconnectedness for the vulnerable and a sense of being cared for. It is the 'humanness' that is highly valued by patients in the UK, but one that needs monitoring carefully (Levy 2008). Although empathy and compassion may be central to the caring aspects of international healthcare curricula, Shapiro (2008) identifies that there is increasing research evidence that once in practice, medical students are losing this aspect of caring in favour of more distant, powerful approaches.

Table 3.5 Eight domains of care that patients indicated as their highest priorities (Levy 2008)

- Fast access to reliable health advice
- Effective treatment by trusted professionals
- Shared decisions and respect for preferences
- Clear information and support for self-care
- Attention to physical and environmental needs
- Emotional support, empathy and respect
- Involvement of and support for family and carers
- Continuity of care and smooth transitions

According to Patistea (1999), the term 'to care for' is but one of four uses of the word 'care' used within the wider healthcare literature, the remainder being 'to have care of, to care about and to care that' (p. 490). Patistea cites Barnum (1998) and Blustein (1991), who identify the term 'to care for' as 'an obvious psychosocial orientation of care and caring'. It is this orientation to care, that, although a strong attribute in the nurse–patient relationship, may not be as strong for physicians whose priority of care is the physical well-being of the patient. It is this Western model of medicine that is currently under criticism (Shapiro, 2008; Youngson, 2008).

Moore (2000) identified that this psychosocial understanding enabled nurses to speak confidently of the patients' feelings and fears, but this was not always well received by doctors. Noddings (1984) found that women in general tend to 'give reasons for their acts, but their reasons point to feelings, needs, situational conditions, and their sense of personal ideal rather than universal principles and their application' (p. 96). These findings may suggest that, when nurses took on the role of advocacy for vulnerable patients, they relayed the feelings and the explicit situation to doctors who, in these cases, interpreted the nurses' position as being too emotional. Moore (2000) noted that in some cases this engendered the emotion of anger in nurses, a feeling of emotional distress that prevented them from thinking clearly (LeDoux 1993).

Norvedt (1996) does not support the view that nurses are too involved with their patients, but he recognises that a problem may arise in the future which may compromise the 'interconnectedness' of care in that 'Professionals may have to weaken their sensitivity and obligations to particular patients in order to satisfy policy demands and considerations of justice' (p. 217). It is the ethic of justice which doctors tend to argue from, as opposed to the care ethic that drives nurses, yet a further diversity in caring and a possible tension as there is a 'tie between relationship and responsibility' (Gilligan 1982: 173).

Tschudin (1999) offers more insight into the complexity of healthcare policy when she states that those who move further away from actual care become 'suspicious and fearful of feelings and try to shield practitioners with policies and instructions' (p. 57). If this is the case, there is a threat to both the nurses' and the patients' integrity (Norvedt 1996). If primary nursing has developed a deeper understanding of what nursing is, and of nurses' perceptions of the patients' psychosocial needs, such a threat identified by Norvedt leads one to question further the future of nursing and caring. This may be especially so as some nurses may, in expanding their roles to take on more medical duties, emulate the Western medical model. According to the International Council of Nurses (1997), there are five important values that underpin the future of nursing, namely:

- visionary leadership
- inclusiveness
- flexibility
- partnership
- achievement.

Each one should relate closely with and complement the others. For example, if healthcare staff are to effectively and justly address the rapidly changing health needs of society in the future, there needs to be an environment of trust and openness for patients and professional groups to work together in partnership (Thompson et al. 1994).

At the end stage of life, such requirements may be a need for patients to share any myths, fears and beliefs concerning their imminent death with the person closest to them at that moment. Campbell et al. (1999) argue strongly for the acknowledgement that end of life decisions, especially regarding treatments, should take into consideration what the competent patient considers to be worthwhile. A competent patient would be regarded as one who has the mental capacity to make decisions. This often raises issues of communication within relationships, especially where patients or other professionals seek further information regarding decision-making.

Within the hospital setting, it is often the nurse whom the patient has chosen to discuss fears or preferences with, or to request further information from. Because patients sometimes pose their questions in 'a masked way', the nurse has to actively listen and interpret the message, and in many instances may need to share aspects with other team members (Arend 1998) or take the lead as an advocate. Within community care, it may not be the nurse whom the patient first confides in, but it could be the nurse in charge of the caseload or the case manager who may receive concerns from formal carers and have to advocate in the situation, or in the case of those with mental incapacity, who may need to involve the 'new Independent Mental Capacity Advocate (IMCA) service created under the Act' (Ministry of Justice 2005: 178; DH 2007c).

The role of advocacy is complex and one that should not be undertaken in ignorance (Gates 1994; Teasdale 1998). It is important for nurses to know their limitations and understand the complexities of the advocacy role. Gates (1994) advises that, due to many problems, nurses need 'to separate their professional and employee roles from any potential advocacy role' (p. viii). An example of a problem arising is where nurses have sought to use the patient as a 'pawn' in a power game to raise their professional status (Teasdale 1998; Godsell 1999).

Teasdale (1998) also suggests that nurses need to read situations carefully because it may at times be easy to 'get caught up in the emotional outrage at the ways in which patients are treated or mistreated' (p. 75).

The end stage of life is already an emotional time for many, so it is important for healthcare professionals to be able to read situations and identify risks within roles, any moral problems and ways of addressing them.

Support for vulnerable patients who believe they may need help with managing their private goods and making decisions regarding health can now be arranged through an LPA. EPA is still valid, but new applications will be the LPA. The LPA differs from the EPA in that it can be registered with the Public Guardian at any time before or after the person (donor) lacks the capacity to make decisions. It also covers more differences (see the Ministry of Justice 2005). There will be separate laws to support the EPA and the LPA, but the code advises only on the LPA. In situations where the patient may be extremely vulnerable, such as those diagnosed with dementia, there is protection via the Court of Protection (Ministry of Justice 2005). In the future, the LPA could offer support for patients discharged into the community following a wish to die at home.

Scenario 3.4 suggests a complexity in discharge planning at the end stage of life, especially continuity of care and 'access of services across geographical or sectoral boundaries' (Levy 2008: 33). Levy suggests that there needs to be more focus on public values and an 'integration of the idea of co-production/co-creation of health with patients, with clear shared responsibility for health outcomes' (p. 19). This will challenge traditional professional ways of working, so it will be important for healthcare staff to read situations carefully, identify any moral issues that need attention, share information, be creative and learn to work together.

Scenario 3.4: The complexity of discharging a dying man into the community

A man 63 years of age, who lives in a small border village between two countries in the UK, has recently been diagnosed with an aggressive lung cancer by consultants working in one country. As he has been told that he has weeks to live, the man has said that he would prefer to die at home. He has requested that the preferred narcotic to control his pain should be one that will allow him, as far as possible, to attend to his normal duties at home, such as cooking, fishing, planning his funeral and saying goodbye to trusted friends. Although the consultant, GP and palliative care service come from one country, the district nursing and social care is managed from the other. The consultant prescribes a more expensive narcotic that will allow the man the space to attend to his end of life activities. The GP, however, tries to replace this drug with a cheaper narcotic that will heavily sedate the patient.

> **Reflection points**
>
> - What are the moral issues and problems here, and how can they be resolved?
> - What systems need to be in place to ensure the provision of seamless care and that the patient can die at home?

According to van den Hurk (1991), cited by Arend and Remmers-van den Hurk (1999), many nurses were unable to define the concept of a moral problem. Moore (2000) found that many of the tensions within teams involved 'end of life decision making', and that the nurses were able to define the problem, but needed to be more articulate and confident in discussing new ways of working with conflict within a team. Time is required to explore any moral issues with teams, and it is by reflecting and exploring that practitioners can improve their confidence to act (Benner 1984).

Many have argued that tensions at this stage of life can marginalise patients and effect poor outcomes (Heenan 1990; Stein et al. 1990; Keddy et al. 1986). Moore (2000) found that the greatest tensions for nurses were in situations where doctors were seen to be making decisions in isolation, not listening or willing to discuss issues with other team members or, in many cases, with the patient and informal carers. In a situation where there was lack of consultation, Tschudin (1999) would raise a concern that 'moral truths are not taken into consideration' (p. 69). Within Moore's study, the nurses often expressed a feeling of not being valued, that their opinions or those of the patients did not matter as the doctor gave the impression that he or she knew best. These are situations that appear to be common, for as The (1997), cited by Arend (1998), and Moore (1999) found, nurses often felt that doctors did not take them seriously.

Tschudin (1999) argues that in healthcare the 'vision' should be 'the ethical stance that people matter' whether they are patients or team members (p. 110). At the end stage of life, Arend (1998) acknowledges the value of nurses' expertise and involvement in the psychosocial care of the patient. In Moore's (2000) study, there was one example of inclusiveness where, after the patient's death, a nurse was included in a debriefing session. Such an example is one that could be shared within teams as a positive and powerful critical incident from which others could learn (Benner 1984).

Arend (1998) cites the work of The (1997), who identified that, in some cases, nurses and physicians do not regard one another as colleagues but 'obstacles to overcome before their own targets can be realised'

(Arend 1998: 316). It may be that, in the Dutch example, the physician was using an avoidance of the need to discuss what had happened as a coping strategy for what might have been a distressing situation that was compromising his beliefs, and one which he was unable to handle effectively. The coping strategy allowed him to reach his target of hiding true feelings of inadequacy. By remaining aloof and in some way in denial of a limitation in his practice, the physician might have been disadvantaging not just the patient, but also the rest of the team and the family unit (Moore 2000).

Another possibility is that the doctor may believe he 'knows best', and that he regards himself as the leader of the team. This is a traditional view of leadership, which still exists today in many countries. An example is sadly apparent in some of the electronic responses to Leavitt's (2000) observations of the interplay between a doctor and nurse in the emergency room – a situation where the nurse was 'quietly in control of the situation', organising, supporting, leading and thinking ahead, while the doctor was perceived as asserting her superiority, regarding the nurse as the 'little helper' when it was obvious that it was the doctor who had limitations. An angry response by Khan (2000) reiterated the belief that doctors should be superior and the natural leaders of the team. Such an attitude does little to promote a learning environment or support a learning organisation, a vision which has support at the macro level of policy-making in Britain (DOH 2000b, 2000c). According to Senge (1990: 359), the learners within such an organisation are in fact the 'natural leaders' who will eventually 'provide a framework for focusing the effort to develop the capacity to lead', a vision contrasting with that of Khan (2000).

A question arises here of what abilities these 'natural leaders' should have to achieve such a goal. Senge (1990) identifies these as 'an ability to develop conceptual and communication skills, to reflect on personal values, and to align personal behaviour with values, to learn how to listen and to appreciate others and others' ideas' (pp. 359–60). Such abilities are enabled through the learning disciplines of systems thinking, personal mastery, mental models, building shared visions and team learning, which, Senge (1990) argues, could also be called leadership disciplines.

Time to experience and reflect on the leadership disciplines and the qualities and diversities of the team may be just the therapy that is required to start to build a collaborative team. Within healthcare, it could be argued that the building of a shared vision of caring should be led by a collaborative team of professionals, each realising mutual trust and respect (Johns 1999; Tschudin 1999), respect, that is, of the need for team decision-making and for time to consider the power of reflection for the team (Lipp 1998).

While these diversities and tensions of care are best explored and valued within teams, there is still the diversity between the ethics of justice and the ethics of care that needs to be addressed if harmony within a multi-disciplinary team is to be achieved and patient participation is respected. The NMC standards (2008) do emphasise that healthcare professionals have a 'shared set of values,' which 'are reflected in the different codes of each of the UK's healthcare regulators' (p. 7). This statement and the content of the new standards reflect the principles of the Human Rights Act 1998, the Mental Health Act 2007 and the draft revised Mental Health Act Code of Practice (2007). At the macro level of policy-making, there is now evidence of some joined-up thinking and working. The challenge for the future will be for practitioners, patients and policy-makers at local levels to work together to enable the embedding of the principles to enhance quality of care.

Nurses working in the community will face a bigger challenge as the profile of nursing expands and crosses professional boundaries, and the expectations of patients accessing a growing number of healthcare amenities will become more demanding. A central value for the nurse working with the daily tensions and diversities of caring in the community must be a respect for, and belief in, humanity. Space to reflect and share concerns with colleagues and patients, and a plan to resolve issues must be important features of practice in today's modern, hectic world.

Conclusion

This chapter has explored some paradigm shifts in healthcare that underpin the need for change and the need for health and social care staff to respect the cultural perspectives, ethical stances and values of patients and families. The scenarios are real stories, although names have been changed, and permission has been given for their inclusion to aid practitioners to reflect and learn.

New ethical issues will arise as patients, carers and practitioners engaged in health and social care become more familiar with the Human Rights Act 1998, and the voice of the patient becomes more prominent in effecting change. Therefore, it is important for health and social care teams to consider how they can learn with patients and plan for change without losing the compassion and empathy of caring. Bigger ethical issues, especially those affecting the end stage of life, in particular for older people, will challenge traditional ways of thinking and working, as well as personal values and beliefs. Time to explore and debate the bigger ethical issues and tensions will be a work-based challenge, but one that could be so valuable in ensuring the respect of individuals and their rights, not just for the patient, but for all involved in healthcare. It is time to share such values and ease the tensions.

References

Arend, A.J.G. (1998) An ethical perspective on euthanasia and assisted suicide in the Netherlands from a nursing point of view. *Nursing Ethics* 5(4): 307–18.

Arend, A.J.G. and Remmers-van den Hurk, C.H.M. (1999) Moral problems among Dutch nurses: a survey, *Nursing Ethics* 6(6): 468–82.

Beauchamp, T. and Childress, J. (2001) *Principles of Biomedical Ethics*, 5th edn. New York: Oxford University Press.

Benner, P. (1984) *From Novice to Expert: Excellence and Power in Clinical Nursing*. Menlo Park, CA: Addison-Wesley.

British Medical Association (1995) *Advance Statements about Medical Treatment: Code of Practice with Explanatory Notes*. London: BMA.

Burnard, P. and Chapman, C.M. (1988) *Professional and Ethical Issues in Nursing*. New York: John Wiley & Sons.

Campbell, A., Charlesworth, M., Gillett, G. and Jones, G. (1999) *Medical Ethics*, 2nd edn. Oxford: Oxford University Press.

Chester, M. (2000) *Human Rights Issues*. London: Association of Community Health Councils for England and Wales.

Chinn, P.L. (1995) *Peace and Power: Creating Community for the Future*, 4th edn. New York: National League for Nursing.

Curtin L. and Flaherty, M.J. (1982) *Nursing Ethics: Theories and Pragmatics*. Washington: Prentice Hall International.

Department of Health (2000a) *The Vital Connection: An Equalities Framework for the NHS*. Available from http://www.dh.gov.uk/en/Publicationsandstatistics/Publications/PublicationsPolicyAndGuidance/DH_4007652.

Department of Health (2000b) *The NHS Plan: A Plan for Investment, a Plan for Reform*. Available from http://www.dh.gov.uk/en/Publicationsandstatistics/Publications/PublicationsPolicyandGuidance/DH_4002960.

Department of Health (2000c) *Meeting the Challenge: A Strategy for the Allied Health Professions*. Available from http://www.dh.gov.uk/en/Publicationsandstatistics/Publications/PublicationsPolicyAndGuidance/DH_4025477.

Department of Health (2005) *Supporting People with Long Term Conditions: An NHS and Social Care model to Support Local Innovation and Integration*. Available from http://www.dh.gov.uk/en/Publicationsandstatistics/Publications/PublicationsPolicyAndGuidance/DH_4100252.

Department of Health (2006a) *Our Health, Our Care, Our Say: A New Direction for Community Services*. Available from http://www.dh.gov.uk/en/Publicationsandstatistics/Publications/PublicationsPolicyAndGuidance/DH_4127453.

Department of Health (2006b) *The Expert Patients Programme*. Available from http://www.dh.gov.uk/en/Aboutus/MinistersandDepartmentLeaders/ChiefMedicalOfficer/ProgressOnPolicy/ProgressBrowsableDocument/DH_4102757.

Department of Health (2007a) *Human Rights in Healthcare – a Framework for Local Action*. Available from http://www.dh.gov.uk/en/Publicationsandstatistics/Publications/PublicationsPolicyAndGuidance/DH_073473.

Department of Health (2007b) *Mental Health: Draft Revised Code of Practice and Secondary Legislation.* Available from http://www.dh.gov.uk/en/Healthcare/NationalServiceFrameworks/Mentalhealth/DH_079861.

Department of Health (2007c) *Making Decisions: The Independent Mental Capacity Advocate (IMCA) Service.* Available from http://www.dh.gov.uk/en/Publicationsandstatistics/Publications/PublicationsPolicyAndGuidance/DH_073932.

Dimond, B. (1997) *Legal Aspects of Care in the Community.* Basingstoke: Macmillan.

Dworkin, R. (1977) *Taking Rights Seriously.* London: Duckworth.

Dworkin, R. (1990) *A Bill of Rights for Britain.* Counterblasts No. 16. London: Chatto and Windus.

Fry, S.T. (1994) *Ethics in Nursing Practice: A Guide to Ethical Decision Making.* Geneva: International Council of Nurses.

Gates, B. (1994) *Advocacy: A Nurses' Guide.* London: Scutari Press.

Gilligan, C. (1982) *In a Different Voice.* Cambridge: MA Harvard University Press.

Godsell, M. (1999) *Caring for People with Learning Disabilities.* In G. Wilkinson and M. Miers (eds) *Power and Nursing Practice.* London: Macmillan.

Hancock, C. (2000) Introduction. In R. Wilkinson and H. Caulfield, *The Human Rights Act: A Practical Guide for Nurses.* London: Whurr.

Harris, J. (1987) QALYifing the value of life. *Journal of Medical Ethics* 13: 117–23.

Healy, P. (2001) Share deal. *Nursing Standard* 15(1): 17–18.

Heenan, A. (1990) Playing patients. *Nursing Times* 86(46): 46–8.

Hek, G. (1998) *Ethical Issues in Community Health Care District Nursing.* In R. Chadwick and M. Levitt (eds) *Ethical Issues in Community Health Care.* London: Arnold.

House of Commons Health Committee (2004) *Elder Abuse, 2nd Report of Session 2003–2004,* Vol. 1. London: HMSO.

House of Lords Select Committee on Medical Ethics (1994) *Report, Paper 21-I.* London: HMSO.

Hudson, A.J. and Moore, L.J. (2006) A new way of caring for older people in the community. *Nursing Standard* 20(46): 40–7.

International Council of Nurses (1997) ICN plans for nursing's future directions, News, 11 January, ICN/97/3.

Illich, I. (1987) *Disabling Professions.* London: Marian Boyars.

Johns, C. (1999) Unravelling the dilemmas within everyday nursing practice. *Nursing Ethics* 6(4): 287–95.

Keddy, B., Gillis, M.J., Jacobs, P., Burton, H. and Rogers, M. (1986) The doctor–nurse relationship: an historical perspective, Canada in the 1920's and/or 1930's. *Journal of Advanced Nursing* 11(6): 745–53.

Kennedy, I. (2001) *Learning from Bristol: The Report of the Public Inquiry into Children's Heart Surgery at the Bristol Royal Infirmary 1984–1995.* CM 5207. Available from http://www.bristol-inquiry.org.uk/.

Khan, M.B. (2000) An electronic response to Leavitt's article in the *British Medical Journal.* Available from http://www.bmj.com/cgi/eletters/321/7276/1621#EL2.

Kohner, N. (1996) *The Moral Maze of Practice.* London: King's Fund.

Kuhn, T.S. (1970) *The Structure of Scientific Revolutions.* Chicago: Chicago University Press.

La Fontaine, J., Ahuja, J., Bradbury, N.M., Phillips, S. and Oyebode, J.R. (2007) Understanding dementia amongst people in minority ethnic and cultural groups. *Journal of Advanced Nursing* 60(6): 605–14.

Leavitt, F. (2000) Garages and hospitals, doctors and nurses. *British Medical Journal* 321: 1621.

LeDoux, J.E. (1993) Emotional memory systems in the brain. Behavioural Brain Research 58(1–2): 69–79.

Levy, D.A.L. (2008) *An Independent NHS: What's in it for Patients and Citizens?* Report for the Picker Institute Europe. Available from http://www.pickereurope.org/Filestore/Publications/Picker_Independent_NHS_Lo_web.pdf.

Lipp, A. (1998) An enquiry into a combined approach for nursing ethics. *Nursing Ethics* 5(2): 122–38.

McLean, S. (1996) End-of-life decisions and the law. *Journal of Medical Ethics* 22: 261–62.

Maynard, A. (1987) Logic in medicine: an economic perspective. *British Journal of Medicine* 295: 1537–41.

Miller, C., Ross, N. and Freeman, M. (1999) *The Role of Collaborative/Shared Learning in Pre-and Post Registration Education in Nursing, Midwifery and Health Visiting.* Research Highlights No. 39. London: ENB.

Ministry of Justice (2005) *Mental Capacity Act 2005 Code of Practice.* Available from http://www.justice.gov.uk/docs/mca-cp.pdf.

Moore, L.J. (1999) *Advanced Directives: Empowering Nurses to Journey through the Ethico-legal Minefield of the End-stage of Life Decisions.* Unpublished report presented at the International Council of Nurses Centennial Congress, London.

Moore, L.J. (2000) *Empowering Health Care Professionals to Support Patients' Rights at the End Stage of Life.* London: Florence Nightingale Foundation.

Moore, L.J. (2007) Partnerships and work-based learning: an evaluation of an opportunity to pioneer new ways to care for the older people in the community. *Assessment and Evaluation in Higher Education* 32(1): 61–77.

National Institute for Health and Clinical Excellence (2006) *Supporting People with Dementia and their Carers in Health and Social Care.* Clinical Guideline No. 42. Available from http://www.nice.org.uk/nicemedia/pdf/CG042NICE-Guideline.pdf.

Noddings, N. (1984) *Caring: A Feminine Approach to Ethics and Moral Education.* Berkeley, CA: University of California.

Norvedt, P. (1996) *Sensitive Judgement.* Oslo: Tano Aschehoug.

Nozick, R. (1974) *Anarchy, State and Utopia.* London: Basil Blackwell.

Nursing and Midwifery Council (2006) *A–Z advice Sheet: Consent.* Available from http://www.nmc-uk.org/aDisplayDocument.aspx?DocumentID=2893.

Nursing and Midwifery Council (2008) *The Code – Standards of Conduct, Performance and Ethics for Nurses and Midwives.* Available from http://www.nmc-uk.org/aArticle.aspx?ArticleID=3057.

Nyberg, D. (1981) *Power over Power*. Ithaca, NY: Cornell University.

Office of Public Sector Information (2007) *Mental Health Act 2007*. Available from http://www.opsi.gov.uk/acts/acts2007/ukpga_20070012_en_1.

Office of Public Sector Information (1998) *Human Rights Act 1998*. http://www.opsi.gov.uk/ACTS/acts1998/ukpga_19980042_en_1.

O'Keeffe, M., Hills, A., Doyle, M. et al. (2007) *UK Study of Abuse and Neglect of Older People, Prevalence Survey Report*. London: National Centre for Social Research, King's College.

Paine, T. (1987) *Rights of Man*. New York: Prometheus Books.

Patistea, E. (1999) Nurses' perceptions of caring as documented in theory and research. *Journal of Clinical Nursing* 8(5): 487–95.

Rawls, J. (1973) *A Theory of Justice*. Oxford: Oxford University Press.

Rawls, J. (1989) Castigating QALY's. *Journal of Medical Ethics* 15: 143–7.

Rokeach, M. (1969) *Beliefs, Attitudes, and Values*. San Francisco: Jossey-Bass.

Royal College of Nursing (2005) *Appraisal Consultation Document Regarding the Review of Alzheimer's Disease Drugs by the National Institute of Clinical Evidence*. Available from http://www.nice.org.uk/nicemedia/pdf/AD_ER_CCACD_RCN.pdf.

Seedhouse, D. (1988) *Ethics: The Heart of Healthcare*. London: John Wiley & Sons.

Senge, P.M. (1990) *The Fifth Discipline: The Art and Practice of the Learning Organisations*. London: Century Business.

Shapiro, J. (2008) Walking a mile in their patients' shoes: empathy and othering in medical students' education. *Philosophy, Ethics, and Humanities in Medicine* 3: 10.

Smith, J. (2005) *The Shipman Inquiry, Final Report*. Available from http://www.the-shipman-inquiry.org.uk/.

Stein, L. Watts, D. and Howell, T. (1990) The doctor–nurse game revisited. *New England Journal of Medicine* 322(8): 546–9.

Stephenson, J. and Weil, S. (1992) *Quality in Learning: A Capability Approach in Higher Education*. London: Kogan Page.

Teasdale, K. (1998) *Advocacy in Health Care*. Oxford: Blackwell.

Thompson, I.E., Melia, K.M. and Boyd, K.M. (1994) *Nursing Ethics*, 3rd edn. Edinburgh: Churchill Livingstone.

Thompson, M. (2005). *Ethical Theory*, 2nd edn. Abingdon: Hodder Murray.

Tschudin, V. (1999) *Nurses Matter: Reclaiming our Professional Identity*. Basingstoke: Macmillan.

Veatch, R.M. (1981). *A Theory of Medical Ethics*. New York: Basic Books.

Waldron, J. (ed.) (1987) *Nonsense on Stilts*. London: Methuen.

Wenger, E., McDermott, R. and Snyder, W.M. (2002) *Cultivating Communities of Practice*. Boston: Harvard Business School Press.

Wile, R., Postle, K., Steiner, A. and Walsh, B. (2003) Nurse-led intermediate care: patients' perceptions. *International Journal of Nursing Studies* 40(1): 61–71.

Wilkinson, R. and Caulfield, H. (2000) *The Human Rights Act: A Practical Guide for Nurses*. London: Whurr.

Williams, A. (1985) The value of QALY's. *Health and Social Service Journal* 95: 3–5.

Youngson, R. (2008) *Compassion in Healthcare: The Missing Dimension of Healthcare Reform?* Futures Debate. London: NHS Confederation.

Section 2
Contemporary challenges

Chapter 4

Healthy ageing, active ageing: the challenges

Angela Hudson, Jane Buswell and Natalie Godfrey

Introduction

The biomedical model of age is one that ties ill-health and impairment to old age in a way that defines ageing as an inevitable and thereby an untreatable process of physical and mental decline (Bytheway et al. 2007). The focus of health promotion for older adults has normally focused on specific disease prevention strategies – stroke, falls and coronary heart disease (*National Service Framework for Older People*; Department of Health [DH] 2001); however the economic drivers of reducing hospital admissions of older adults (Hudson and Moore 2006) have not taken into account the multiple social and environmental factors that can adversely affect the health of older adults.

The focus of prevention of disease has always been at the forefront of public health in the UK, particularly since the pioneering work of Edwin Chadwick (1800–90), who, as Sanitation Commissioner in Victorian England, campaigned for changes in the law to include the reform of sanitation, education and transportation. In 1854, Surgeon John Snow (1813–58) removed the handle of a drinking pump infected by leakage from a sewer and stopped an outbreak of cholera. These two men made a substantial contribution to public health in Victorian Britain, particularly to the health of the working classes and the resultant increase in longevity.

In 1901, Joseph Rowntree recognised that older people were at increased risk of poverty. Jones and Sidell (1997) have confirmed that poverty, socio-economic status and ill-health are closely linked. Given these stated facts, any attempts at health promotion and education must encompass an holistic approach that considers the structural inequalities in society (Benzeval et al. 1997), rather than focusing on an individual's lifestyle (Mechanic 1999). This has particular implications for any health-promoting activity with older people, given their vulnerable position within society.

This chapter explores the concept of healthy and active ageing, and considers the challenges to overcome in relation to older people. It will examine current models of health promotion and their relevance for the older person. The challenges to active ageing will be explored, with attention given to barriers and attitudes to healthy ageing. Finally, contemporary and hidden health issues for older people will be considered in relation to sexual health, alcohol and substance misuse, and depression and suicide.

The context

As the UK's population ages, the number of older people with one or more long-term conditions (LTCs) is set to increase, and the cost to the National Health Service (NHS) of treating this increased caseload could be unaffordable. The current shift in the UK is towards self-management of LTCs. Keeping people healthy in spite of the disabilities experienced with LTCs is an important political driver. There are an estimated 17.5 million people with an LTC in the UK (DH 2005b), which covers the entire lifespan from 0 to 100 years. As discussed in Chapter 2, life expectancy has in recent years increased, i.e. people are living longer. England has the highest and Scotland the lowest life expectancies at birth of the home nations.

Three-quarters of older people live with at least one LTC, the most common of which is arthritis, particularly in women, and cardiovascular disease in men. A total of 42% of men and 41% of women report that their LTC limits their daily living activities (Age Concern 2008). Up to 25% of older people living in the community have symptoms of depression that warrant intervention and that affect their quality of life (Age Concern 2007a). This is discussed later in this chapter.

Given this information, it is evident that LTC management consumes a large part of NHS resources – about 80% of GP consultations and 60% of hospital bed days (DH 2005b, 2008). In fact, just 2% of patients with an LTC account for 30% of emergency hospital admissions, and 10% of inpatients with LTC account for over 50% of hospital bed days. However, these statistics focus on the comparatively small number of people with multiple LTCs whose conditions are unstable and complex. The NHS and social care LTC model (often referred to as the 'Kaiser triangle') would place these individuals at Level 3 (Box 4.1). Of the 17.5 million people with an LTC, it is estimated that there are just 5% at Level 3. What will be of primary importance over the next decade is ensuring that health and social care professionals work with older people at Levels 1 and 2 in order to maintain healthy and active lifestyles and prevent progression to level 3.

Box 4.1 Levels of care – National Health Service and social care long-term conditions model (Department of Health 2005)

Level 3 – 5% of the population with long-term conditions with highly complex needs, for whom case management is the recommended model. These patients are managed by a case manager, advanced primary nurse or community matron

Level 2 – 20–25% of the population with long-term conditions. These are high-risk patients for whom disease management is the recommended model of care. These individuals could be managed by a disease-specific specialist nurse, e.g. diabetes nurse specialist or other professional such as a physiotherapist with specialist knowledge. They could be managed by a community nursing team. The aim is to ensure these individuals do not move to Level 3 care

Level 1 – 70–80% of the population with long-term conditions, for whom self-management is suitable. These individuals could also be supported to maintain health and well-being by assistant practitioners or workers such as health trainers. (Health trainers are unqualified individuals who give advice and support regarding, for example, exercise regime, lifestyle change and dietary advice)

Underpinned by health promotion – population wide

In Box 4.1, we can see that underpinning the three levels of care is a focus on health promotion with 'whole' populations. Community health and social care professionals are in a prime position to facilitate this and provide appropriately targeted health promotion and education for older people that considers both primary prevention (such as immunisation) and secondary prevention (such as cardiac rehabilitation). However, health promotion activities can sometimes be misjudged or misapplied to older adults. Scenario 4.1 is an example of this.

Scenario 4.1: A misjudged cardiac rehabilitation programme

Annie is 82 and has had a myocardial infarction. During her hospital, stay a zealous physiotherapist visits her as part of the hospital's cardiac rehabilitation programme. One of the activities she is asked to do is to climb a flight of stairs to increase her physical activity and reduce the risks of further infarctions. Annie protests, and explains she has osteoarthritis of her knees and hips that limits her mobility. The physiotherapist insists that stairs must be done before Annie can go home. Annie tries to climb the stairs but has great difficulty because of the osteoarthritis. The physiotherapist has read this information in Annie's notes and assumed that she could 'kill two birds with one stone' and improve Annie's restricted mobility from her osteoarthritis. Annie gets very upset and distressed, and telephones her daughter, who informs the physiotherapist that Annie has no need to climb stairs as she lives in a bungalow and has not climbed stairs for the last 30 years.

Reflection points

- How could this situation have been avoided?
- What activities could the physiotherapist have suggested as an alternative to stair-climbing that are more age specific?

As discussed more fully in Chapter 2, the population of the UK is an ageing one that has resulted largely from a decline in mortality and birth rates and advancements in technology. The current population of older people in the UK varies widely from those just entering old age, that is, the first of the so-called 'Baby Boomers' (those born between 1946 and 1964) and those born prior to the First and Second World Wars, i.e. pre 1900–1945. This gap of some 48 years poses unique challenges for health professionals (World Health Organization [WHO] 2006) in terms of focused targeting of health information and activities to a cohort whose ages could range from over 100 down to 60 years of age. Additionally, health and lifestyle issues impact on the ageing UK population in different ways.

Expectations of health between cohorts of older people will vary greatly and be influenced by social and economic forces and life experiences. For the current cohort of older people, technological advances in healthcare and improved post-war living conditions mean that many older people are living longer. However, these extra years are not always spent in good health, and as Soule et al.'s (2005) report on the 2001 census indicates, the percentage of over 65s who report having a long-standing illness or chronic ill health is 60% for men and 65% for women. This has implications in terms of health expenditure as a significant proportion of the current spending on health and care services is attributed to older adults (DH 2008). Improving health promotion among this group of the population may have economic benefits, but for older people in particular it can maintain their health and well-being, providing them with the opportunity to be as disability free as possible.

For the 'Baby Boomers', maintaining a healthy lifestyle is viewed as a normal part of everyday life, and this cohort have been subject to a wide range of health promotion messages and high-profile campaigns through their lifespan, such as the Smoking Kills campaign. The increasing use of the Internet has meant there is a wealth of information easily and quickly available about how to stay healthy and where to get help and advice on staying active as one ages. It will be important therefore that healthy and active ageing activities and programmes consider this heterogeneous group of people. Although the benefits of smoking cessation and a diet low in saturated fats and added salt could be applied across the older-person age range, it is clear that some activities and programmes need more careful targeting in order to achieve maximum benefit for the older person and an improved quality of life that adds life to years rather than years to life.

Active ageing

Active ageing is a continuous adaptive process (Mayhew 2005). Since health and well-being in older age are largely a result of experiences throughout the lifespan, our biological systems such as muscle strength and cardiac function reach their peak in early adulthood and then decline. How quickly this happens is determined by external factors relating to lifestyle, including smoking, alcohol consumption, diet and socio-economic status. The Organisation for Economic Cooperation and Development (1998: 84) defines active ageing as:

> the capacity of people, as they grow older, to lead productive lives in the society and the economy. This means that they can make flexible choices in the way they spend time over life – in learning, in work, in leisure and in care-giving.

Active ageing applies to physical, social and mental well-being throughout the life course, participating in society on a social, economic, cultural and spiritual level (WHO 2008). The WHO (2008: 1) defines active ageing as:

the process of optimising opportunities for health, participation and security in order to enhance quality of life as people age. It applies to both individuals and population groups.

Although the individual may not have control over early life experiences and other factors such as poverty or low education, actions taken during the remaining life-course greatly affect health in later life.

Healthy ageing

Hansen-Kyle (2005: 52) offers the following definition of healthy ageing:

Healthy ageing is the process of slowing down, physically and cognitively, while resiliently adapting and compensating in order to optimally function and participate in all areas of one's life (physical, cognitive, social, and spiritual).

An alternative definition is provided by Healthy Ageing – A Challenge for Europe, a 3-year (2004–07) project co-funded by the European Commission that aimed to promote healthy ageing among people aged 50 years and over:

the process of optimising opportunities for physical, social and mental health to enable older people to take an active part in society without discrimination and to enjoy an independent and good quality of life. (Swedish National Institute of Health 2007: 5)

What these definitions highlight is that healthy and active ageing is about making choices, about adding life to years rather than years to life, and about empowering older people to achieve optimum outcomes in terms of health and lifestyle. Older people may, however, encounter obstacles to achieving healthy active ageing. These barriers include ageist assumptions and attitudes, and socio-economic and structural barriers.

Barriers

A range of intrinsic and extrinsic barriers exist for the older person in relation to physical activity. Intrinsic barriers relate to the beliefs, motives and experiences of the individual (British Heart Foundation 1999) and could relate to previous experience, safety concerns (traffic, fear of attack, and slips, trips and falls) and lack of confidence (embarrassment or anxiety). Extrinsic barriers relate to the broader environment, for example the attitudes of others and recreation policies, which may prevent older people joining or maintaining a new activity. It is generally accepted that age discrimination should be rooted out wherever it occurs (Mayhew 2005), yet ageism continues to exist and provides a barrier to many activities (AGE 2004).

Older people need to be consulted in the planning of activity programmes so that barriers can be identified and addressed (Young 1996). Financial cost, insufficient time and the lack of culturally appropriate facilities also act as barriers, although these are not specific to older people. Activity programmes and class design affect participation by older people (British Heart Foundation 1999). The level of difficulty, instructor competence and cost and timing of sessions are important considerations to promote inclusion.

For older people, Finch (1997) and Rai and Finch (1997) have identified age-specific barriers such as:

- fears about 'overdoing it' – concerns about overexertion 'at their age', particularly for those with medical problems
- practical safety concerns – cold water, slippery swimming pool edges or a fear of falling during exercise
- traffic near the class, and fear of attack
- health professional and family advice – '. . . at your age?'
- myths and perceptions – what is and what isn't good.

Evandrou (2005) reported that membership of a sports club, gym or exercise class for women at ages 65–69 was 23%, as opposed to 19% for men at the same age. Activities such as swimming, bowls, ballroom dancing, walking and tai chi are all activities that are less strenuous than gym work but would contribute to both physical and mental health and well-being in the older person.

Attitudes

Ageist assumptions regarding the needs of older adults in maintaining their health and well-being remain embedded in many areas of practice, and persist in many older people themselves, for example:

- Older people will not want or need to be in peak health – if they're not in paid employment, what else have they got to do?
- Health problems are 'just your age'
- Older people are less interested in preventative measures to safeguard their health
- Older people will (or will not) want specific treatments or services without asking for them.

Attitudes are ingrained through stereotyping. People are influenced by how older people are portrayed in the media and in society (Mayhew 2005). Stereotypes may be positive or negative, but are generally distortions of fact. The Seniors Network (2008) list 23 common stereotypes or myths, one of which is 'that the majority of older people view themselves as being in poor health' (p. 1). Within the media, images of older people are rarely positive (AGE 2004), and old age is often presented as a time of physical, mental and social decline (Redfern and Ross 2006). Given these perceptions, it is no surprise that ageist attitudes persist and that health promotion and education activities are not targeted at the older age group. For governments, primary care trusts, acute trusts and other organisations, the ageist practice of rationing care and treatment on the basis of age continues covertly, despite assurances to the contrary. Breast screening is a good example of this.

Breast screening

The apparent contradiction in promoting active healthy ageing may be illustrated by the current UK programme for breast cancer screening. Current evidence indicates that the risk of breast cancer increases with age, and that it is important that women continue with regular screening as this has been shown to reduce risks (Advisory Committee on Breast Cancer Screening 2006). Since 1988, the NHS has provided free 3-yearly breast screening for all women in the UK aged 50 and over. Once women reach their 70th birthday, however, they are no longer routinely invited to attend; instead they are encouraged to make their own appointments.

The aim of breast cancer screening is to reduce the number of premature deaths, and the evidence is that it is achieving its aim. The rationale of issuing a blanket invitation is to proactively offer a defined at risk population the opportunity to be screened, reminding them of the health risks and benefits of screening and giving them an informed choice, leaving older women free to opt out of screening rather than to opt in. The premise that if someone is in good health but not judged to have a life expectancy of more than 10 years is, it could be argued, fundamentally ageist (Bytheway et al. 2007).

Socio-environmental barriers

Access to transport is vital for older adults if they are to participate in activities in their community. For some, private transport is accessible, although at the age of 70, and then 3-yearly thereafter, driving licence renewal is required. Those older adults who rely on public transport face challenges as many transport services are not designed with older people in mind (Help the Aged 2008). The use of community transport services such as Dial-A-Ride, voluntary or charity organisations buses allows older people with mobility problems the opportunity to participate more actively. Often, however, knowledge of these services is not widespread, and community nursing staff will be in a position to advise older people on what is available.

Many older people look for support to stay in their own homes, in the form of services and equipment in order to maintain health. Yet many continue to live in poverty even though they are entitled to claim assistance. In 2007 4 billion pounds in benefits remained unclaimed by older adults. Reasons attributed to this were related to poor advertising, different benefits having different criteria and end means-testing, which made older people feel uneasy about divulging their personal and financial details (Help the Aged 2008). The cost of attending clubs, social activities and sporting clubs could be severely hampered by a lack of funds to participate, further increasing the older person's isolation and limiting their attempts to remain active.

Older people may feel afraid to leave their homes in order to seek out social opportunities or health activities. They may be afraid about crime, 'no-go' areas and being subject to attacks, either verbal or physical. Again, the community nurse can help alleviate these concerns by providing the older person with information, support and encouragement.

It is clear that older people are disadvantaged because of structural inequalities, such as reliance on public transport, a poor standard of housing and reduced social networks (Victor 2000). The changing face of the geographical landscape is also an important consideration. Many local shops have been replaced by out of town supermarkets that may have an extensive choice but are inaccessible to many older people because of mobility problems or the distance from home. Therefore, the ability to eat healthily, for example, may be affected not just by the accessibility and availability of the goods, but also by other extrinsic factors that need to be considered when evaluating the success of any health promotion programme (Andrews 2001).

Policy frameworks

A plethora of policies, strategies and initiatives are currently driving the UK health and social care agenda, aimed at reducing the rising economic costs of supporting older adults with ill-health and moving away from the purely biomedical focus on acknowledging the impact of social isolation. One of the difficulties in considering any policy document is that, for the four countries of the UK, policies will differ in both their expectation and their application to their local population. Chapter 2 explored a number of these policies in relation to England and their impact on the older person, and we shall not repeat these here. Nevertheless, a closer examination of policy indicates some common themes, which, if we link them to the three levels of health promotion and education mentioned below (Table 4.1), indicates areas of responsibility for nurses at an individual level:

- population-wide macro level, for example immunisation
- local and community based, such as exercise classes
- individual micro level – personalised programmes.

Table 4.1 Common themes through older person policy linked with three levels of health education/promotion

Theme	Level
Promoting independence and mobility	Macro, local and individual
Engaging and consulting with older people	Macro and local
Improving and integrating services	Local
Social inclusion and addressing health inequalities	Macro and local
Developing strategic partnerships	Macro and local
Preventing ill-health, disease and disability	Local and individual
Preventing accidents among older people	Macro, local and individual

Health promotion versus health education

Whitehead (2004) explores the differences between health promotion and health education, and notes that the use of a reductionist approach in health promotion activities, i.e. focusing on reducing the incidence of specific disease or reducing the burden of ill-health, continues to be the favoured approach. Indeed, it could be argued that the philosophy of Standard 8 of the National Service Framework is a reductionist one, in that despite Philp's (2002) assertion to the contrary, the focus is on disease rather than socio-economic and structural factors (Young 1996).

Health education on the other hand focuses on a behaviour change (Mechanic 1999, Whitehead 2001), uses an approach that is beneficent in nature, to the extreme point of paternalism (Seedhouse 1995; Buchanan 2000), and tends to be considered separately from the more global notion of health promotion. However, the terms appear to be used interchangeably throughout the literature, and it is apparent that health promotion activities or targets do not have a clearly defined trajectory, and therefore, as Victor (2000) confirms, health promotion for older people lacks a clear definition and purpose. Speller et al. (1998) confirms that the lack of consensus about the nature, purpose and efficacy of health promotion may lead to indifference on the part of health professionals.

Traditional models of health promotion focus on convincing individuals to behave in a different way to improve their disease trajectory. More contemporary models recognise the importance of negotiation with individuals to empower them to make adjustments to their lifestyles, and these models also consider that individuals are influenced by communities, and that social empowerment is as important as individual behavioural change. In this respect, the concept of social marketing has expanded and is an area of rapidly developing growth, particularly in relation to health behaviour. It is 'the systematic application of marketing concepts and techniques, to achieve specific behavioural goals to improve health and reduce health inequalities' (French and Blair-Stevens 2006: 2).

Health-related social marketing has three key features:

1. 'Its primary aim is to achieve a particular 'social good' (rather than commercial benefit) with specific behavioural goals clearly identified and targeted.
2. It is a systematic process phased to address short, medium and long-term issues.
3. It utilises a range of marketing techniques and approaches (a marketing mix). In the case of health-related social marketing, the 'social good' can be articulated in terms of achieving specific, achievable and manageable behaviour goals, relevant to improving health and reducing health inequalities.' (National Social Marketing Centre 2006)

Models of health promotion

Health promotion is a process of enabling people to increase control over their health and its determinants, thereby improving their health (National Cancer Institute [NCI] 2005; WHO 2006). It is guided by a set of principles that are common to a number of other disciplines, such as public health, primary healthcare, community development and environmental health (Redfern and Ross 2006). The practice of health promotion is underpinned by a number of theories and models. A theory is an abstract integrated set of propositions that explains a phenomenon, examples of which are social cognitive theory (Bandura 1986) and the theory of planned behaviour (Ajzen 1985). Models are a subclass of a theory and may draw on a number of other theories to help understand a context-specific problem; the transtheoretical model (Prochaska and Di Clemente 1983) and the health belief model (Glanz et al 2002) are two such examples. Health promotion programme planning, implementation and monitoring processes that are based in theory are more likely to succeed than those developed without a theoretical perspective (NCI 2005). We shall consider how these models might apply to the older person.

Transtheoretical (stages of change) model

The basic premise of the transtheoretical (stages of change) model (Prochaska and Di Clemente 1983) is that behaviour change is a process rather than an event, during which the individual moves through five stages (Lach et al. 2004; Prochaska et al. 2006): precontemplation, contemplation, preparation, action and maintenance:

- *Precontemplation* is where an individual has no intention of changing behaviour, due to either resistance or an inability to see the problem
- *Contemplation* relates to the individual's awareness, where change is being considered in the next 6 months. Although the individual may be receptive to information at this stage, the desire to change may not be sufficient. It is possible to remain at this stage for many years.
- *Preparation* is where active planning takes place, or small steps are taken to make the change within the next month.
- *Action* is where individuals are engaged in the changed behaviour for less than 6 months
- *Maintenance* is where the individual has successfully changed behaviour and maintained it for longer than 6 months.

These stages may be achieved in a linear fashion, or the individual may move back and forth repeating stages (Lach et al. 2004). The focus of this model is the individual's readiness to change or attempt to change toward healthy behaviours (Health Promotion Agency 2005).

The informational needs and change strategies deployed differ at each stage (NCI 2005). At the precontemplation stage, personalised information about risks and benefits to raise awareness of the need for change would be employed, whereas at the action stage, assistance with feedback, problem-solving, social support and reinforcement strategies are required. Although this model originated from studies in smoking cessation, it has been applied to many others (Reicherter and Greene 2005), including addiction (Davidson 1992; Chilvers et al. 2002). It has also been successfully incorporated into a range of older adult health promotion programmes (Nigg et al. 1999; Burbank and Riebe 2002; Lach et al. 2004).

The health belief model

The health belief model is one of the most widely recognised models in the field of health promotion and has been used since its development in the 1950s. It is a psychological model that attempts to explain and predict health behaviours by examining the influences on individual's decisions about whether to take action to prevent, screen for and control illness (NCI 2005). It considers individuals' perceptions of susceptibility, severity, benefits and barriers, as well as cues to action and self-efficacy. It has been applied to a broad range of health behaviours and populations in preventative health, health risk and sick role behaviours (University of Twente 2004). As health motivation is the central focus of health belief model, it is suited to addressing behaviours such as high-risk sexual behaviour and the resulting possibility of contracting human immuno-deficiency virus (HIV; NCI 2005). In terms of the older person, this model may be useful as it relies on understanding individuals' beliefs about their health.

The precaution adoption process model (PAPM)

The precaution adoption process model (Weinstein 1988) applies to behaviours that require intentional action and can help to explain why and how people make deliberate choices. It has seven stages that map out the individual's journey from awareness to action (Blalock and DeVellis 1998). It has been applied to osteoporosis prevention, colorectal cancer screening and mammography (NCI 2005).

Targeted health education for older people

As people are living longer, health promotion activities are of increasing importance and can provide years of benefit, by adding years to life. Yet with the reported variables in terms of older adults' engagement in these activities (Resnick 2003), individualised approaches are required. Young (1996) asserts that older people welcome health promotion activities if provided in easily accessible forms, and that many people over the age of 75 already engage in activities designed to maintain or improve their health (Scenario 4.2). Glass et al.'s (1999) study demonstrated that the survival of older people is improved by participation in a range of social and leisure activities.

Scenario 4.2: 50+ Healthy Living – Bristol City Council

In 2007, Bristol City Council's Celebrating Age Festival included a 2-week programme aimed at the over 50s of over 70 sport and fitness sessions at local leisure centres, sports centres and pools across the city for free or at a substantially reduced fee. The council's web pages include a 50+ healthy living page that aims to:

- promote health and well-being in Bristol
- focus on all the sectors of Bristol's community, thus reducing health inequalities.

Links are included to Active Choices, a physical activity referral programme, and a University of Bristol Community Exercise programme. This is an example of information effectively targeting the older age group (Bristol City Council 2007).

Reflection points

- **Reflect on any health promotion/health education activities available in your local area that are specifically targeted at older people.**
- **What are the activities, and are they accessible in terms of venue, access, cost and availability?**

The traditional and core methods of health promotion – i.e. behaviour change – may be less appropriate in older people because of structural inequalities in the system. Older people may be excluded from adopting healthy practices and lifestyles and health promotion activities. Additionally, many older people (especially women) are disadvantaged by their reliance on public transport and reduced social networks.

Katz et al. (2000) indicate that material and economic disadvantage accumulates over the lifespan, and that poor health in later life cannot be corrected by what Speller et al. (1998) label the 'one shot approach' to improving health. In interviews with older people, Young (1996) elicited that issues such as finance, transport and housing were as important to health as good physical status.

Challenges

Lay beliefs

Older people's lay beliefs are also important to consider when exploring the value of certain activities (Parry et al. 2002). There is, however, some ambiguity about the type or focus of health promoting activities for older people. Wright and Bramwell's (2001) study on skin cancer highlighted the importance of targeting health promoting activities at the right group, and in a way that older people can relate to. The authors make the point that the current cohort of older people believe in the therapeutic effects of the sun, and that this is related to their lay beliefs about the positive effects of sunshine on skin. This could stem from a lack of publicity about skin cancer in the 1950s, and also from the lived experience of smog and rickets, both of which were prevalent in the 1940s and 50s before the Clean Air Act of 1956. The importance of lay beliefs is further highlighted by Wright and Bramwell who acknowledged in their study that older people thought skin cancer only affected younger people, and that it was self-inflicted through such activities as sunbathing and sunbed treatments. Campaigns to increase older people's awareness of the development of skin cancer need to consider that many older people think changes in skin pigmentation could be attributed to the normal ageing processes.

Additionally, understanding of the damaging cumulative effects of the sun also needs to increase among older people, as this is one area that has seen an increase in cases in the older age group. This highlights the need for targeted education that is sensitive to the cohorts' health issues of the time. The wholesale approach to health promotion clearly has deficits, as Wright and Bramwell (2001) discovered, in that older people do not see the relevance of the current skin cancer campaign to them. It should also be noted that, with each successive cohort of older people, campaigns and targeted information needs to take account of the changing interests and knowledge of older people. The 'Baby Boomers' of the 1960s (Evandrou 1997) will be a group of people with increased awareness of health damaging activities (such as sunbed use) compared with the cohort of older people of the pre-Second World War era.

On a similar theme, Parry et al. (2002) examined smoking practices in older people and found that, for today's current cohort of older people, smoking was a socially acceptable activity in the 1930s and 40s, the link between smoking and lung cancer would not have been clearly identified until the 1950s (Parry et al. 2002). Despite recent publicity, older people still continue to smoke, perhaps because they have already reached old age and current campaigns tend to focus on people under 65 (Arber 1996; Arcury et al. 2001; Kerr et al. 2002).

Complementary therapies

Ernst and White's (2000) report of a BBC Survey of complementary and alternative medicine (CAM) use in the UK identified that:

- of 166 people over the age of 65 surveyed, 11% had used CAM in the previous year
- of 617 people aged 35–64, 26% had used CAM in the last year.

A study by Wellman et al. (2001) found that 20% of CAM users were over the age of 55 years, with a high proportion represented by the early 'Baby Boomers' (those now aged 60 or over). Clearly, the implications are that these users of CAM will become older users in the next decade with differing health needs and may well increase their usage of CAM. The most popular CAMs (Zollman and Vickers 1999) are:

- acupuncture
- chiropractic
- healing therapies
- herbalism, including Chinese medicine
- homeopathy,
- hypnotherapy
- manual therapies
- reflexology
- naturopathy
- osteopathy.

The reasons given for older people's use of CAM relate to dissatisfaction with standard (known as orthodox) medicine, preventative measures such as warding off colds, holistic care, an increased amount of one-to-one time and support; relaxation and the relief of symptoms of LTCs, particularly pain. In Andrews' (2002) study of 144 users of CAM, 42% were aged 70–79. In these older users, the most common condition for which CAMs were utilised were musculoskeletal, which accounted for 59% of all conditions. We need to be cognisant of the fact that some older people's use of CAM predates the creation of the NHS in 1947, and therefore the use of CAM may be considered as an empowering process of managing their own health. The return to more traditional and natural remedies such as manuka honey for leg ulcers has been greeted with enthusiasm by many older people, eager to use a remedy that does not contain ingredients that could have side-effects.

However, there are two major difficulties that older people may experience in their continued use of CAM. One is cost, and the other is regulation and legitimacy of the CAM practitioner. At present, anyone can set themselves up as a CAM practitioner without regulation. The exceptions to this are chiropractors and osteopaths, who have statutory self-regulation in place and protection in regard to their titles. This means that these titles are protected by law, and only people qualified with the regulatory bodies are allowed to practise. Acupuncture and herbal medicine are the next CAM practitioners awaiting regulation. For older people, the abundance of CAM practitioners advertising their services can be overwhelming, and it would be difficult to distinguish and determine who is the most appropriate practitioner. Older people may look towards health practitioners, nurses in particular, to suggest a practitioner or give advice. The Prince's Foundation for Integrated Health and the Complementary and Natural Healthcare Council (established in April 2008) have informative websites that provide guidance and advice on CAM. The NHS *Directory of Complementary and Alternative Practitioners* has a website that allows a search for a therapist in the local area, as does SAGA. Age Concern has a useful book with information about the different types of complementary therapy, and Help the Aged has excellent information on CAM and finding a practitioner.

Ernst and White's (2000) report of the BBC survey identified that 29% of CAM users in the 65 and over age group spent from £11 to £35 per month on treatment modalities. This compares with just 2% spending over £35. However, there are a number of therapies available on the NHS. Most commonly these are homeopathy, osteopathy and acupuncture. The GP surgery should have a list of locally available therapies, and the GP should be able to refer the older person to the appropriate CAM practitioner. As a health practitioner, it is important to share this information with the older person in order for them to avoid unnecessary expenditure. It is also important for the health professional to provide information for the older person to make an informed choice about the therapies available.

Controversy and cultural shifts

This next section considers three areas of health that are considered challenging and require a cultural shift of thinking in older person practice. Sexual health, alcohol and substance misuse, and depression and suicide are three subjects that nurses find challenging and difficult to tackle in practice, particularly in the community setting.

Sexual health for older adults

For many older adults, ageing brings increased confidence and sexual awareness and becoming comfortable with their bodies. Laurance (2008) reported on a Swedish study of sexual activity in those over 70, which highlighted that 'Those who were in their thirties during the sexual revolution of the 1960s still retain a liberal attitude to sex four decades later' (p. 1). The report also identified that the number of older men and women continuing to have sex into old age had increased, from 52% to 68% in men and from 38% to 56% in women.

This, however, contrasts with the ingrained ageism of our society in which older people are stereotyped as being non-sexual beings who should not, cannot and do not want to have sex. A report by the Research on Age Discrimination Project (Bytheway et al. 2007) highlighted that 47% of people surveyed agreed that society discourages older people from expressing themselves sexually. Health, not age, determines the level of sexual satisfaction in older people's lives. A recent US study reported that sexual activity drops only slightly from the 50s to the early 70s; thereafter, declining health is matched by a corresponding fall in the frequency of love-making. Many men and women remain sexually active until well into their 70s and 80s (Lindau et al. 2007).

Diana Athill, a 90-year-writer, editor and publisher recently, commented: 'the most obvious thing about moving into my 70s was the disappearance of what was the most important thing in life: I ceased to be a sexual being' (Athill 2008).

In the UK, older adults who participated in a Help the Aged study (Bytheway et al. 2007) commented: 'Older people aren't supposed to want sex and there is little help with problems such as erectile dysfunction or dry vaginas, and of course you can't be on hormone replacement therapy in the UK if you are 65' (p. 58). Interviewees described encounters in which health professionals automatically assumed individuals were sexually inactive and were embarrassed to ask about sex, even where it was directly relevant to the treatment offered, such as that for prostatic cancer or diabetes. Bytheway et al. (2007) comment that:

> Doctors rarely discuss sex with older patients, social workers fail to look at older people's sexual histories or needs when assessing them and service providers fail to take account of sexuality in planning the care and support they offer to older people. (p. 57)

For the older person in the community, the significance of remaining in a caring and fulfilling relationship is important, particularly for those who have been in long-term relationships (Sabin 1993).

Although sexual drive and intensity diminish in later life, evidence indicates that while penetrative sex remains important, other forms of sexual and sensual satisfaction become increasingly significant (Vincent et al. 2000). The need for intimacy continues whatever the age, and community nurses must consider this aspect in their care and treatment plans. If a bed needs to be brought downstairs for increasing care requirements, it is crucial that the nurse suggests or is able to facilitate ways in which the older person and his or her long-term partner can continue with intimate aspects of their relationship. This could be very simple suggestions, such as ensuring equipment is unobtrusive and kept to a minimum, giving assisting with personal grooming and the application of make-up, to allowing space on the bed for a couple to cuddle and share intimacy. Masturbation and oral sex can be a helpful way for older people who are incapacitated by LTCs to achieve satisfaction and intimacy with or without a partner (Kellett 1993). The use of sex aids such as vibrators can help older women achieve sexual pleasure (Scenario 4.3). Community nurses need to ensure that older people have access to information about safe sex and positioning, ways to achieve sexual satisfaction such as using vibrators and other sex aids, and where to get the aids, particularly if the older person does not have access to the Internet. The community nurse should also know how and where to refer onto for specialist help with sexual dysfunction.

Scenario 4.3: Sexual health

Mary is 82 and lives alone. She has become more disabled over the last 5 years as she now has advanced osteoarthritis in her knees and hips, which she finds affects her mobility. Mary has a community nurse visit once a week to dress her leg ulcers with four-layer bandaging. They often share a joke and repartee about men and bodies, and Mary points out which men she fancies off the TV. On one of the visits, Mary starts discussing vibrators, as she has read in a magazine that many women use them to achieve sexual pleasure. She wonders if the community nurse knows where she can buy one. The community nurse is rather taken aback by this request, and is uncomfortable that Mary is discussing such matters openly and frankly. She brushes Mary off by saying that she doesn't think this is a subject Mary should be discussing. Mary is mortified by the community nurse's response as she believed that the community nurse would be able to discuss these issues without embarrassment.

Reflection points

- How would you feel in this situation?
- How would you approach the issue, and what advice could you give Mary in order to answer her question?

For older people in care homes, the maintenance of intimate and sexual relationships is challenging. Bytheway et al. (2007) comments on this in the *Too Old* report:

> Two panel members referred to the way social care agencies sometimes dismiss long-standing relationships by separating couples when one of them needs residential care. This raises the question of how far such decisions are prompted by ageist assumptions about sexual inactivity. (p. 58)

Moving into a care setting can have a profound impact on relationships and the ability to continue a sexually intimate relationship. Lack of privacy, with regimented institutional practices, can abruptly terminate intimate relationships. Trying to find space for intimacy in a care home can be challenging when the resident may share that space with other people (Scenario 4.4). The older person's life may also have been disrupted by the move to a care home. For many, this is a traumatic and distressing time, precisely when they may need physical contact and comfort most, and their sense of self and their relationships may be adversely affected. Szasz (1983) conducted a survey exploring nursing home staff attitudes towards acceptable sexual behaviour. The staff responses were that hugging and kissing were the only acceptable and (they implied) the only *permitted* forms of such behaviour.

Residents who masturbate in public areas can cause distress and discomfort to staff and other residents, and it is often perceived as a 'behaviour problem' rather than a need to express their sexuality, relieve frustration or tension or feel comforted (White 2001). Care home staff need to be cognisant of the need for privacy and dignity to allow older people the opportunity to sexually express themselves.

Scenario 4.4: Tensions

John and Julia have been together 57 years. Julia is in a care home, and John manages to visit her once a month. On each visit, John takes Julia to her bedroom, and asks staff to ensure they are not disturbed. John has even made a 'Do Not Disturb' notice for the bedroom door. The staff of the care home are very concerned by this behaviour and have asked John to conduct his visits in the public spaces, where he can be observed. John is very upset and angry about this and has refused. He has stated he has a right to spend time with his wife sharing private moments.

Reflection points

- How would you tackle this situation?
- Do you think the care home staff have a right to ask John not to spend time with his wife alone? You may wish to refer back to Chapter 3 and the discussion on rights to help you.

Allowing privacy during visits of spouses or partners should be considered good practice. It is recognised, however, that there may be tensions in allowing these intimate visits, particularly if there is concern regarding the nature of the relationship if one partner is a vulnerable adult. In this situation, nurses should conduct a risk assessment that examines the relationship and clearly outlines if there are any concerns. These concerns should be openly discussed among the wider team, documented and discussed with the resident, the partner and the multidisciplinary team.

Despite the older person's confidence how do we as nurses begin to broach the subject? It can be difficult to ask someone with much greater life experience questions relating to the most intimate aspects of their life. Nurses can be as much as four generations younger than the older person they are working with, which can compromise constructive professional discussion. However, nurses need to normalise questions about sexual practices in much the same way as they discuss other intimate aspects of life such as bowel care. Duffin (2008) highlights the fact that the ideal opportunity for nurses to discuss sexual health practices is when they are performing cervical smears or discussing continence or bowel problems or how to increase exercise. Sex is a great way to exercise and improves sleep (Persson 1980). If questions about sexual health are discussed in a 'matter of fact', ordinary way, older people and health professionals will feel less embarrassed about not just the questions, but also the answers.

Sexual dysfunction in older adults

Sexual dysfunction may have a physiological or a psychological basis. The most common problem is fear of or actual impotence. This is the diminished effectiveness or frequency of sexual activity, or a diminished or absent erectile response. In men, there are a range of factors that can contribute to sexual dysfunction:

- reduced hormone levels
- cardiac disease
- pain

- diabetes
- arthritis of back, hips and knees
- excess alcohol
- physical trauma
- prostate disease.

Medications such as antidepressants, beta-blockers, analgesics and anti-hypertensives can reduce desire and arousal and affect erectile dysfunction. Medications may interfere with the capacity of the penis to become erect or ejaculate. This increases with age (Feldman et al. 1994), with approximately 25% of men aged 65–74 years and 75% of men over the age of 85 years experiencing impotence. Erectile dysfunction is more common in men with diabetes, with an increased likelihood (up to 95%) of men over the age of 70 experiencing difficulties with erectile function (Diabetes UK 2008).

Treatment for erectile dysfunction

Vacuum erectile devices and implantable prostheses work by engorging the penis and making it sufficiently stiff to allow penetration (Heath and Schofield 1999). Sildenafil (Viagra) and tadalafil work in part by dilating the blood vessels; however, when combined with other vasodilators such as nitrates taken for angina or chest pain, there are potentially dangerous side-effects, especially for older men, as the additive effect can cause plummeting blood pressure, myocardial infarctions or cerebrovascular events. Polypharmacy, common in older adults, can lead to problems. Tagamet, diltiazem, verapamil and erythromycin can all interfere with the body's ability to metabolise Viagra. Men who have diabetes or coronary heart disease, or have had strokes, and wish to take Viagra should discuss this with their GP. About 25% of men over the age of 65 are prescribed Viagra, and it is recommended that they commence on half the normal dose. When reviewing medication, be sure to ascertain that no over-the-counter (OTC) medications are being taken alongside prescribed drugs, and be aware that Viagra can be bought off the Internet.

The most common sexual problems for women aged over 60 include vaginal dryness, dyspareunia and loss of libido, symptoms usually triggered by the onset of menopause. Women could also experience vaginal prolapse and incontinence, which will affect their body image and their sexuality. An organisation such as Women's Health Concern (see Useful websites at the end of the chapter) has a helpline with dedicated nurse counsellors who can help women with these symptoms. Its website provides some good advice and information for health professionals, and there are downloadable fact sheets on a range of topics including vaginal dryness and sex after the menopause.

Sexually transmitted infections

Despite their absence from the formal policies and strategies, it is evident that older people have contributed to the rise in sexually transmitted infections in the UK. The *Guardian* newspaper (McVeigh 2001) reported that, in the UK, gonorrhoea and syphilis have increased by 55 % since 1995; in the 65 and over age group, the rise is more than 300%. Data from the USA indicate that 11% of all new AIDS cases are in people over 50. In a survey undertaken by researchers from City University, 11% of 1700 people surveyed with HIV were over 50 and 2.6% were over 60 (Duffin 2008). Promoting safe sex is essential with older people as well as those in younger age groups. One of the challenges for health promoters will be to ensure that advice regarding safe sex is not just focused at the under 25s. Older people are just as likely to have casual sex but are less likely to discuss it openly (Rogstad and Bignell 1991).

Relationship issues

Many older gay, lesbian and bisexual (GLB) adults have reported it harder to access support than heterosexual people, both formally and informally (Bytheway et al. 2007). In interviews with older gay men, Bytheway et al. reported that they talked of living through the period when homosexuality was criminalised. Heaphy et al. (2003) provided evidence of the resilience of the older person in relation to the significant risks (often of violence and harassment) that being open about one's sexuality can entail.

This is an important influence on lifestyle and experience, and the impact of attitudes towards ageing and sexuality has specific implications for the 'invisibility' of older lesbians and gay men. Knowledge that an older person may be gay, lesbian or bisexual is often met with negative reactions or ignored, particularly when an older person may be experiencing bereavement and the assumption is made that the relationship is an heterosexual one. GLB older people also have difficulties in meeting other partners and, as Heaphy et al. (2003) reported, this has implications for day-to-day support and care in times of crises; in addition, few had made plans for unexpected health events.

In Heaphy et al.'s study, the participants broadly shared the view that older GLB individuals are discriminated against and socially excluded from society. Opportunities for social networking are often limited. Social support networks, clubs, dating agencies and singles bars are set up for younger GLBs; older people are not encouraged to join or welcomed openly. The younger GLB community discriminate against the older GLB population by perpetrating such descriptions in advertisements such as 'no dirty old men' and 'no wrinklies allowed'. To combat this, Age Concern have provided a comprehensive list of links to GLB support networks and other areas of interest specifically for older GLB individuals. There are a range of fact sheets available, including one with advice on how to 'come out' to a health professional. Age Concern also offer training on GLB ageing issues. In addition, they also support Voice and Choice courses specifically geared to improving the skills of older people so they can more effectively express their opinions around such difficult issues.

For transgender (trans – an umbrella term covering transsexuals, transvestites and those who have undergone gender reassignment) older people, Age Concern (2007b) have provided an excellent fact sheet on planning for later life including information on gender reassignment. This can be undertaken on older people in their 60s, 70s and 80s. Each case should be considered on its merits, but the older trans individual may find that surgery is restricted to people under the age of 65. This is another example of where age discrimination can be effected. The experience of being trans will be dependent on the age at which this occurred. If it happened in their 20s, the older person will have had different experiences from those of someone who has recently transitioned.

As a trans ages, he or she may find that relationships, particularly sexual relationships, are more difficult to sustain. It may have been difficult or impossible to fashion a penis for female to male trans individuals if they had surgery in the 1960s or 70s as surgical techniques were not as advanced as they are today. Male to female trans may experience vaginal dryness or soreness, as well as dyspareunia.

Alcohol and substance misuse

Substance misuse

In the UK, little is known about problematic drug use among older people, probably because they represent a 'hidden' population (Shah and Fountain 2008), and because, as Phillips and Katz (2001) comment, the nature and pattern of substance misuse in older people differs from that in younger people. Shah and Fountain (2008) offer a number of explanations for their underidentification:

1. Criminal activity is positively correlated with problem drug use (particularly opiates), and there are a lower proportion of older offenders
2. Older people are less likely to acquire illegal drugs through the street drug scene
3. A decline in social function may not be attributed to problem drug use but to changes associated with ageing

4. Cognitive impairment may not be attributed to problem drug use but to changes associated with ageing
5. Signs of problem drug use may mimic physical disorders
6. There may be a lack of awareness of medical and nursing staff that problem drug use may be an issue.

'Substance misuse' is a term used to describe harmful use and dependence. Substances can be prescribed or illegal and include alcohol and tobacco. Harmful use is classed by the 10th revision of the WHO's *International Classification of Diseases* (WHO 1990) as causing functional impairment related to changes in lifestyle at school, work or home. Immediately we can see that this classification may cause some serious difficulties in identifying problematic substance use in the older person as they may have an altered lifestyle (perhaps due to retirement from paid work) and some degree of functional and cognitive impairment that may not be related to substance misuse. The classification of dependence relates to behaviour such as increased tolerance of use, more use of income to buy substances and withdrawal symptoms.

The scale of problematic drug use among older people is relatively unknown (Phillips and Katz 2001), although Beynon et al. (2007) report in their study in Cheshire and Merseyside, an increase in numbers over 8 years. For example, the number of male problematic drug users aged 50–74 in contact with agency-based syringe exchange programmes in the area between 1998 and 2004 increased from 24 to 65. Although these numbers are small compared with those under 50 years of age, estimates indicate that by 2025 more than 25% of the UK's population will be over 60 years old, and this generation will have grown up in a period when illicit drug use was more prevalent.

Statistics available for the older population are limited, but the prevalence of drug dependence in Great Britain within the 65–69 age group is reported (McGrath et al. 2005) to be:

- 4 per 1000 population for tranquillisers
- 7 per 1000 adult population for cannabis

and that within the 70–74 years age group to be:

- 1 per 1000 for tranquillisers
- 4 per 1000 adult population for cannabis.

The most misused substances are prescribed drugs and OTC medicines. Beynon et al. (2007) found that older users combined OTC medications, prescribed medicines and alcohol, resulting in physiological and psychological changes that could be falsely attributed to the ageing process or side-effects from prescribed medicines. Within the older population, many clinical conditions mimic substance misuse, and hence misdiagnosis is almost unavoidable (McGrath et al. 2005). Healthcare professionals will therefore need to be vigilant and consider substance misuse if an older person presents with falls, an unexplained or unexpected increase in drowsiness, depression, insomnia or confusion. Community nurses and other staff who are prescribers will need to be thorough with their history-taking and consider the potential for an older person to be drug dependent.

Strachan (2001) identified that, in the UK, older people receive 45% of all written prescriptions. McGrath et al. (2005) further noted that older people tend to have multiple drug regimens of at least five prescribed medicines, hoard medicines and use OTC medicines in conjunction with prescribed medicines without any knowledge and understanding of their interactions. Misuse of sedatives is high in this age group, and older people are far more likely than younger people to be prescribed benzodiazepines. In addition, older people may take more than the prescribed dosage of medication. Side-effects may be increased as the ageing liver and kidney cannot metabolise medications quickly, and there maybe a build-up of medications in the body. This may result in drowsiness, falls and confusion. Any older person with these signs should have a medication review, remembering that it is not just prescribed medicines that need reviewing.

Prescription and OTC drugs are used widely by older adults. Around one third of all prescribed drugs, which often include benzodiazepines and opioid analgesics, are used by people aged over 65 years. The misuse of prescribed or OTC drugs may involve deliberately using higher than recommended doses, 'borrowing' a medication from a friend or relative, use for extended periods, hoarding medications and using medications together with alcohol. This may lead to persistent and problematic use and dependence. Often drug reactions in older people are complex and unusual, and older people do not always present with standard and uniform signs of adverse reactions.

Benzodiazepines are most commonly prescribed for anxiety in older people, particularly older women (Currie 2004). Cheng et al. (2008) identified that benzodiazepines could be used by as much as 42% of older people in the community. Their usage continues because they are extremely cheap (around 6 p for 20 tablets at the time of publication) compared with more effective medications such as Prozac (around £21 for 30 tablets). Benzodiazepines can impair cognitive functioning, memory and balance at therapeutic dose levels, and because they are often prescribed for longer than the recommended time period (a maximum of 2–4 weeks), older people are at risk of dependence and addiction (Cheng et al. 2008). Benzodiazepine use in older people is associated with an increase of as much as 44% in the risk of hip fracture and night falls (Todd and Skelton 2004).

Table 4.2 Commonly used benzodiazepines

Generic name	Brand or common name
Chlordiazepoxide	Librium
Diazepam	Valium
Lorazepam	Ativan
Oxazepam	
Nitrazepam	Mogadon
Loprazolam	
Temazepam	
Clonazepam	Rivotril
Triazolam	Halcion

Withdrawal symptoms from benzodiazepines include mild delirium tremens, sleeplessness, jumpiness, intense anxiety and panic attacks. Women are more at risk of developing dependency than men. The fact that benzodiazepines are legitimately prescribed makes the detection of dependency and problematic drug use more difficult. Table 4.2 lists the common benzodiazepines prescribed for older people in the UK.

The number of older people requiring treatment for a substance use disorder is likely to more than double between 2001 and 2020 (Gossop and Moos 2008). This is due partly to the size of the 'Baby Boomer' cohort and the higher rate of substance misuse among this group, There is concern that, as the 'Baby Boomers' age, the demand for substance-use treatment will increase substantially (Gfroerer et al. 2002). Community staff will need to be aware that substance misuse is a growing problem, particularly in relation to the continued and increased usage of antidepressants, anxiolytics and benzodiazepines.

Reflection points

- Think about the older people you have recently visited. Did you complete a medication review? Did you ask about *all* medications, including OTC, prescribed and homeopathic remedies?

Alcohol misuse

Like substance misuse, alcohol misuse is underestimated and under-reported due to reluctance to take alcohol histories and because of ageist assumptions that older people do not drink. It is a rapidly developing but poorly understood phenomenon (Phillips and Katz 2001). The identification of alcohol misuse in older people is problematical as older people do not always present with overt indication of alcohol misuse. The belief that older people will be drinking vast quantities of alcohol and are therefore easily identifiable is misleading. It is an underrecognised problem within the UK particularly for health and social care workers (Alcohol Concern 2002).

- *Late-onset alcoholism* is defined as a condition in which people start drinking after 60 years of age and experience one or more symptoms of alcohol dependence; it often occurs as a reaction to a specific life event such as bereavement (Cowart and Sutherland 1998)
- *Early-onset alcoholism* is defined as a condition in which an older drinker continues to consume alcohol, and has done so from an earlier age (Lakhani 1997).

Consumption

The amount of alcohol consumed daily or weekly is often considered a reliable way of identifying those individuals who are consuming alcohol at a hazardous or harmful level (Box 4.2). The recommended weekly limits of 21 standard units for men and 14 standard units for women (Clough et al. 2004) are a recognised benchmark in the UK for identification of overconsumption but have not changed for the past 20 years (Alcohol Education and Research Council 2005). However, as Clough et al. identify, many older people do not drink at levels perceived as problematic,

---

Box 4.2 Definitions (WHO 2004)

Alcohol abuse: involves a preoccupation with alcohol and an impaired sense of control over alcohol consumption. Individuals often continue to abuse alcohol despite serious health, personal, work-related and financial problems

Alcohol dependence: people drinking above sensible levels and experiencing harm and symptoms of dependence

Alcoholism: can be defined as the physical dependence on alcohol over a period of time

Harmful drinking: alcohol consumption that results in consequences to physical and mental health and possible social consequences

Hazardous drinking: a pattern of alcohol consumption that increases the risk of harmful consequences for the user or others. Hazardous drinking patterns are of public health significance despite the absence of any current disorder in the individual user

and this could therefore lead to underdetection of alcohol-related problems (Dyson 2006). In older people, this level of consumption may cause serious deleterious effects as these limits do not take into account the effect of alcohol on the ageing body.

The ambiguity and inaccuracy of the standard unit of measurement of alcohol also presents practitioners working with older people with problems when it comes to assessing for signs of hazardous or harmful alcohol consumption. In addition, it does not assist them in providing appropriate advice to older people about recommended drinking limits.

Effects of alcohol on older people

Relatively small amounts of alcohol consumed by older people can have a deleterious effect on the ageing body (Blow et al. 2004). Due to physiological ageing, older people have an increased sensitivity to and intolerance of alcohol as a result of reduced body mass, a decrease in body water volume and changes in hepatic and renal insufficiency, affecting the absorption, distribution and excretion of alcohol (Blow et al. 2004). Older people reach higher peak alcohol levels at lower levels of use than younger adults, placing them at increased risk of intoxification (Adams et al. 1996). Beullens and Aertgeerts (2004) comment that the amount consumed is not a reliable measure: older people can drink less frequently and consume a smaller amount but still experience significant intoxication. Even modest alcohol use in old age is potentially harmful as it contributes to increased falls, poor memory, mismanagement of medication, inadequate diet and the potential for self-neglect (Clough et al. 2004).

Alcohol-related problems may be misinterpreted as normal consequences of ageing, and problem drinking may be overlooked in older people as it may be masked by co-morbid physical or psychiatric illness, be misdiagnosed (e.g. as depression) or be an atypical presentation (O'Connell et al. 2003). Symptoms such as musculoskeletal pain, insomnia, anxiety, memory disturbance and depression are often misdiagnosed, or undiagnosed, in older people, or are attributed to the effects of ageing and not alcohol use (Kopera-Frye et al. 1999). The likelihood of older people mixing alcohol with prescribed and OTC drugs is a real concern. Alcohol can potentiate the sedative effect of many drugs such as benzodiazepines. We saw earlier in this chapter that benzodiazepines are one of the most commonly prescribed and addictive drugs for older people, so combine this with alcohol and it becomes a considerable risk to health.

Health professionals may not expect older people to be alcohol dependent, or may rationalise their expectation by conceptualising it in the face of deteriorating health. Older people themselves may not disclose their alcohol intake, regarding alcohol consumption as having 'medicinal' properties (Naik and Jones 1994). It is therefore essential to recognise that functional ability and psychological health may be affected by minimal levels of alcohol consumption and may have a deleterious effect on the health and well-being of older people.

Reasons for drinking

Hajat et al. (2004) report that alcohol use declines with increasing age, and this is thought to be due to a reduced opportunity to partake of social drinking as friendships and family relationships change. Retirement may also provide less opportunity to enjoy the social aspects of drinking enjoyed when perhaps mobility was better. Many older people also use alcohol for 'medicinal purposes' or as an appetite stimulant to aid sleep (Khan et al. 2006).

For late-onset drinkers, the greatest indicators for alcohol misuse occur in response to life events such as financial problems, bereavement, loneliness, social isolation and lack of social support (Moos et al. 2004). Deterioration in health and increasing pain, anxiety and boredom are also key indicators. Moos et al. comment that patterns of alcohol consumption in older people are affected by a complex mix of factors, including cultural, socio-economic and historical influences, gender and cohort effects, declining physical and mental health and changes in socialisation patterns as older people age.

Blow et al.'s (2004) research identified that the 'Baby Boomers' are drinking more alcohol than earlier cohorts. The Institute of Alcohol Studies report in 1999 on *Alcohol and the Elderly*, and the Alcohol and Ageing Working Group report (2006) commissioned by the Scottish parliament, outlined a number of reasons for this, including higher levels of disposable income, changes in the licensing laws and the social availability and acceptability of drinking among this group.

In moderation, alcohol consumption can have a positive effect on the older person's quality of life. For the health practitioner, trying to establish the nature and extent of alcohol intake is fraught with difficulty as changes in behaviour and reduced social contact can be attributed to many issues related to ageing, changing social roles and retirement.

Effectiveness of screening tools

The three most common screening tools used to identify problem drinkers (Box 4.3) are:

- CAGE – a four-question tool with an emphasis on dependence
- MAST-G – a questionnaire with 24 weighted yes/no questions and an emphasis on drinking behaviours
- AUDIT – with an emphasis on consumption.

Box 4.3 Alcohol screening tests for older people

- **CAGE** = **C** – Cut down, **A** – Annoyed, **G** – Guilty, **E** – Eye-opener
- **MAST-G** = Michigan Alcoholism Screening Test – Geriatric Version (Blow et al. 1992)
- **AUDIT** = Alcohol Use Disorders Identification Test
- **DPI** = Drinking Problems Index (Finney et al. 1991)

CAGE and AUDIT are available at http://cks.library.nhs.uk/alcohol_problem_drinking/making_a_diagnosis/confirming_diagnosis/cage_questionaire

MAST-G is available at http://www2.alcoholcme.com/?id=1776:14076

DPI is available from http://www.ilr.cornell.edu/smithers/docs/Assessing_Problem_Drinking_in_Older_Workers.pdf

---

CAGE is the frequently recommended screening tool of choice (Philpot et al. 2003) but has low sensitivity in older people (Whelan 2003) because it detects the dependent drinker. AUDIT has not been used in the community setting (Babor et al. 2001) but has been assessed for reliability and validity. However, there are some mixed reviews about its sensitivity and specificity in older people (Beullens and Aertgeerts 2004).

MAST-G, a 24-item questionnaire developed by Blow et al. in 1992, and the DPI, developed by Finney et al. in 1991, are the only screening tests developed specifically for use with older people. MAST-G adapts the questions asked in the MAST questionnaire to reflect the daily life of older people, with questions related mostly to physiological effects rather than how drinking may affect work, social circle and lifestyle. The DPI is a 17-item measure designed to assess drinking problems among older adults with questions that are more relevant to the age group. For example, it contains questions related to isolation and self-neglect and a question related to falls, which are consequences that are more likely to occur as a result of drinking among older adults (Bamberger et al. 2006).

Any tools developed and used with older people should therefore focus on experiences of life stressors and health and well-being rather than the legal and occupational implications of alcohol misuse, which have less relevance for older people. Assessment should consider the trigger factors that might precipitate behaviour change in the older person. Undertaking any form of assessment for alcohol use with older people does at least raise awareness on the part of the practitioner and the older person that this could potentially be a problem (Dyson 2006).

Intervention and treatment

Intervention programmes specifically tailored to the older person are limited. Interventions that consider cognitive behavioural therapy, brief intervention therapy and counselling can, however, be helpful. Contact with other services such as community mental health teams and social work teams will be a good resource. They are likely to have more in-depth knowledge of the treatment plans and community services available. Be aware that many alcohol misuse treatment services have an upper age limit of 65. Community nurses will need to have a good awareness and knowledge of what is available in their local area in order to advise and support the older person and their family appropriately. There are a number of excellent organisations providing information for both alcohol and substance misuse (see the list at the end of the chapter), although these are not specific to the older person:

- *Council for Information on Tranquillisers and Antidepressants* provides information on tranquilliser addiction and has professional counsellors
- *Dry Out Now* provides free advice, a counselling service, information on UK treatment centres and excellent downloadable treatment guidelines
- *Alcoholics Anonymous* website has information on its 12-step recovery programme and local meetings; these are not age limited
- *Down your Drink* is an online programme for people to develop safer drinking habits and is not age limited
- *Alcohol Concern* has good information, fact sheets and advice and is not age limited
- *Help the Aged* have a specific section on health advice related to alcohol particularly for the older person.

Mental health issues

Mental health problems are not a normal and inevitable part of the ageing process. The majority of older people enjoy good mental health and make a valuable contribution to society. It is widely acknowledged that the mental health and well-being of older people has been neglected across the spectrum of promotion, prevention and treatment services (Philp 2004; National Institute for Mental Health in England [NIMHE] 2005; National Institute for Health and Clinical Excellence 2008). In 2005, an Older Peoples Mental Health service development guide entitled *Everybody's Business* (Care Services Improvement Partnership 2005) was launched, its main aims being:

- to improve the skill and competence of staff to enhance the detection and management of mental illness
- to promote mental health as part of healthy ageing
- to secure comprehensive specialist mental health services for older adults, with a particular emphasis on community mental health team memory service and liaison clinics

Depression

Depression is the most common mental health problem among older people, followed by dementia (DH 2005a). One in four people aged 65 and over have depression that is severe enough to impair quality of life. The frequency of depression rises with age, and the condition is more common among people in their 80s and 90s than those in their 70s (Osborn et al. 2003). The underdetection and underdiagnosis of depression in older adults is a significant problem. Misdiagnosis of depression is common, often being confused with dementia. The older adult may have delirium, depression, dementia or a combination of all three. Moriarty (2005) comments that:

> one of the most important issues for older people's mental health is the delays that regularly occur before they are offered support. These happen either because of people's reluctance to seek help or under recognition on the part of professionals. (p. 14)

The causes of depression in old age are complex, with demographic, social and biological factors all being implicated. It is recognised that the cause of depression in older people is often a combination of physical, psychological and social factors (Katona and Shankar, 1999). Causes of depression in older people (Moriarty 2005) are related to:

- bereavement
- financial worries
- an increase in disability or worsening of a disease or LTC
- unresolved pain
- moving home
- separation from friends and family
- poor social support
- loneliness
- lower socio-economic status.

Physical deterioration can be rapid in older people with depression. Given that many older people may already have poor physical health, depression can exacerbate this and make the older person extremely ill.

Tools that can be used to assess depression

A detailed history should be taken to ensure that a timeline of events and symptoms are clearly presented in order to distinguish that the older person is experiencing signs and symptoms of depression. The overview document for the Single Assessment Process includes a simple screening measure for depression.

The *Geriatric Depression Scale* is freely available for practitioners to use (see Useful websites at the end of the chapter). It has been validated in many environments and needs no prior psychiatric knowledge. The original Geriatric Depression Scale was a 30-item questionnaire, which proved time-consuming and challenging for some patients (and staff). Later versions of only 15 questions retain only the most discriminating questions while retaining the validity of the original form. It can be used with healthy or medically ill adults, and with mildly to moderately cognitively impaired older adults.

The score in itself does not provide a diagnosis, but people with a higher score are more likely to have depression. It is not a substitute for a diagnostic interview by a mental health professional. Any score above 5 (Box 4.4) should prompt a further in-depth assessment.

The *Goldberg Anxiety and Depression Scale* (GADS) (Goldberg et al 1988) is an 18-item self-report symptom inventory. The GADS has been used with older people in the community. The GADS score is based on responses of 'yes' or 'no' to nine depression and nine anxiety items, asking how respondents have been feeling in the past month. Anxiety scores of 5 or more or depression scores of 2 or more are considered clinically important (Koloski et al 2008).

Box 4.4 Scoring the Geriatric Depression Scale

Score results
- 0–4 = no depression
- 5–10 = mild depression
- ≥11 = severe depression

Treatments for depression

Addressing the key factors outlined above for triggering mental health problems in old age is also the focus for preventing and treating depression. The difficulty for practitioners is that many of these are overlapping, complex and sometimes not amenable to change (Manthorpe and Illiffe 2005). Focusing on just one factor is unlikely to be helpful, but being able to improve factors such as pain and lack of sleep can be a major factor in alleviating depression and thus reducing risk of suicide. An holistic approach focusing on the whole person and addressing physical as well as emotional and psychological needs should be utilised. Challenging the ageist assumption that the signs of depression in an older adult are part of the normal ageing process and therefore do not require active intervention is a major issue, both for older adults themselves and for health and social care professionals.

Antidepressants are prescribed for depression, and older people generally respond quite well (Mottram et al. 2006). However, the side-effects of many antidepressants can cause much anxiety and distress for older people, who may not wish to continue with the medications. In fact, the side-effects may be so severe that the older person is more distressed by taking the medication than not taking it. A community nurse's role would be to carefully monitor the side-effects and offer support, information and encouragement to the older person.

There are a range of complementary therapies and self-help groups that can assist with lifting mood without the need for medication. Self-help measures such as incorporating more physical exercise into a daily routine or going out to a concert or a film has been shown to help older adults feel more positive. If depression is as a result of a loss or bereavement, counselling may also help. Advice from older people who have been bereaved suggests that keeping busy, taking part in social activities, helping others, social support and being able to talk about the deceased person to others all help in coming to terms with bereavement (Bennett et al. 2002).

Suicide

Each year in the UK, approximately 5000 people, many of them over 65 years, take their own lives. Older people account for between 20% and 25% of all completed suicides even though they comprise only 15% of the population (Baldwin 2002). Men aged 75 and over are a group who are particularly at risk, and depression is the leading cause of suicide in older people. Older people with symptoms of depression are 23 times more likely to take their own lives than those without symptoms (Ross et al. 1990). The Samaritans (see Useful websites at the end of the chapter) have reported that suicide prevention strategies have continued to ignore suicide as a significant risk among older people.

Evidence shows that paying attention to the potential methods of how people commit suicide can be an effective preventative measure (Harwood et al. 2000). Doctors could reduce the prescription of combination analgesics, anxiolytics and antidepressants as drug overdoses are the most common single method of suicide among older people. Hoarding medication is common and not in itself a suicide risk, but a supply of drugs may be a means to suicide, so regular efforts to collect and dispose of unused medication makes sense.

Recognising those at risk

There are a range of clues that an older person could have suicidal intentions; these include negative and morbid thoughts, previous suicide attempts, self-neglect, alcohol misuse and depression. Many of the risk factors previously outlined for depression are also risk factors for suicide, which highlights the need to take depression in older people seriously.

Follow-up services are needed for older people who have attempted suicide and for those who deliberately self-harm. Although crisis lines such as the Samaritans exist in the UK, there is as yet little evidence of whether they are used much by older people. There are specific sources of support for relatives and friends who have been bereaved by suicide, such as Survivors of Bereavement by Suicide and Cruse (see Useful websites at the end of the chapter). More vigilant prescribing and regular medication reviews by community nurses will ensure that the means to commit suicide through overdose is restricted. Use of support mechanisms such as telephone support lines for the isolated older person have proven to be effective in providing monitoring and emotional support (Beeston 2006).

Conclusion

In this chapter, we have considered that healthy and active ageing is of increasing importance to older people and to the community. The population of older people in the UK is increasing, and the number of older people with one or more LTCs is set to rise. Health promotion for older people needs to be targeted and cohort specific, as well as relevant to the changing needs of the ageing population. Sexual health, alcohol and substance misuse, and depression and suicide are three areas considered as being of growing importance. We have not considered here the rise of community action programmes aimed specifically at older people, but there are a number of national programmes such as Ageing Well, run by Age Concern, the National Coalition for Active Ageing (Help the Aged) and Extend – a music and movement programme for the over 60s (see Useful websites at the end of the chapter). Community nurses are in a prime position to engage with these programmes, encouraging older people to take steps forward to maintain active health and well-being in later life.

References

Adams, W., Barry, K. and Fleming, M. (1996) Screening for problem drinking in older primary care patients. *Journal of the American Medical Association* 276(24): 1964–7.

Advisory Committee on Breast Screening (2006) *Screening for Breast Cancer in England*. NHS Breast Screening Programme Publication No 61. Available from http://www.cancerscreening.nhs.uk/breastscreen/.

AGE – The European Older Peoples Platform (2004) *Age Barriers: Older People's Experiences of Discrimination in Access to Goods, Facilities and Services*. Available from http://www.ageconcern.org.uk.

Age Concern (2007a) *Improving Services and Support for Older People with Mental Health Problems. UK Inquiry into Mental health and Well-Being in Later Life*. Available from http://www.mhilli.org/.

Age Concern (2007b) *Planning for Later Life: Transgender People*. Available from www.ageconcern.org.uk.

Age Concern (2008) *The Age Agenda 2008: Public policy and older people*. Available from http://www.ageconcern.org.uk/AgeConcern/Documents/AA_2008_Report.pdf.

Ajzen, I. (1985) From intentions to actions: a theory of planned behaviour. In J. Kuhl and J. Beckham (eds) *Action control: From Cognition to Behaviour*. Heidelberg: Springer.

Alcohol and Ageing Working Group (2006) *Alcohol and Ageing: Is Alcohol a Major Threat to Healthy Ageing for the Baby Boomers?* Edinburgh: Health Scotland.

Alcohol Concern (2002) Alcohol misuse among older people. *Acquire* (Autumn): i–vi.

Alcohol Education and Research Council (2005) *Researching and Developing Alcohol policy*. Available from http://www.aerc.org.uk/documents/pdfs/AERC_Harm_Reduction_Strategy_Response.pdf.

Andrews, G. (2001) Promoting health and function in an ageing population. *British Medical Journal* 322(24): 728–9.

Andrews, G. (2002) Private complementary medicine and older people: service use and user empowerment. *Ageing and Society* 22(3): 343–68.

Arber, S. (1996) Is living longer a cause for celebration? *Health Service Journal* 106(5512) p 28–31.

Arcury, T., Quandt, S. and Bell, R. (2001) Staying healthy: the salience and meaning of health maintenance behaviours among older rural adults in North Carolina. *Social Science and Medicine* 53(11): 1541–56.

Athill, D. (2008) *Somewhere Towards the End*. London: Granta Books.

Babor, T., Higgins-Biddle. J., Saunders, J. and Monteiro, M. (2001) *AUDIT, The Alcohol Use Disorders Identification Test: Guidelines for use in Primary Care*, 2nd edn. Available from http://whqlibdoc.who.int/hq/2001/WHO_MSD_MSB_01.6a.pdf

Baldwin, R.C. (2002) Suicide in older people – can it be prevented? *Reviews in Clinical Gerontology* 11(2): 107–8.

Bamberger, P., Sonnenstuhl, W.J. and Vashdi, D. (2006) Screening older, blue-collar workers for drinking problems: an assessment of the efficacy of the

Drinking Problems Index. *Journal of Occupational Health Psychology* 11(1): 119–34.

Bandura, A. (1986) *Social Foundations of Thought and Action: A Social Cognitive Theory.* Englewood Cliffs, NJ: Prentice Hall.

Beeston, D. (2006) *Older People and Suicide.* Available from http://olderpeoplesmentalhealth.csip.org.uk/silo/files/older-people-and-suicide.doc

Bennett, K.M., Smith, P.T. and Hughes, G.M. (2002) *Older Widow(er)s: Bereavement and Gender Effects on Lifestyle and Participation.* Research Findings 6 from the Growing Older programme. Available from http://www.shef.ac.uk/uni/projects/gop/Bennett_F6.pdf.

Benzeval, M., Judge, K. and Whitehead, M. (1997) Tackling inequalities in health: extracts from the summary. In M. Sidell, L. Jones, J. Katz and A. Peberdy (eds) *Debates and Dilemmas in Promoting Health – a Reader.* Basingstoke: Macmillan.

Beullens, J. and Aertgeerts, B. (2004) Screening for alcohol abuse and dependence in older people using DSM criteria: a review. *Ageing and Mental Health* 8(1): 76–82.

Beynon, C., McVeigh, J. and Roe, B. (2007) Problematic drug use, ageing and older people: trends in the age of drug users in northwest England. *Ageing and Society* 27(6): 799–810.

Blalock, S. and DeVellis, R. (1998) Health salience: reclaiming a concept from the lost and found. *Health Education Research* 13(3): 399–406.

Blow, F., Brower, K.J., Schulenberg, J.E., Demo-Dananberg, L.M., Young, J.P., Beresford, T.P. (1992) The Michigan Alcoholism Screening Test – Geriatric Version (MAST-G): a new elderly-specific screening instrument. *Alcoholism: Clinical and Experimental Research* 16: 372.

Blow, F., Brockman, L. and Barry, K.L. (2004) Role of alcohol in late life suicide. *Alcoholism: Clinical and Experimental Research* 28(5): 48s–56s.

Bristol City Council (2007) *50+ Healthy Living.* Available from http://www.bristol.gov.uk/ccm/content/press-releases/2007/oct/celebrating-age-festival—fun-for-the-over-50s.en.

British Heart Foundation (1999) *Active for Later Life: Promoting Physical Activity with Older People.* Available from http://www.bhf.org.uk/default.aspx.

Buchanan, D. (2000) *An Ethic for Health Promotion –Rethinking the Sources of Human Well Being.* Oxford: Oxford University Press.

Burbank, P. and Riebe, D. (eds) (2002) *Promoting Exercise and Behaviour Change in Older Adults: Interventions with the Transtheoretical Model.* New York: Springer.

Bytheway, B., Ward, R., Holland, C. and Peace, S. (2007) *Too Old: Older People's Accounts of Discrimination, Exclusion and Rejection. A Report from the Research on Age Discrimination Project (RoAD) to Help the Aged.* Available from http://www.open.ac.uk/hsc/research/research-projects/road/the-road-reports.php.

Care Services Improvement Partnership (2005) *Everybody's Business: Integrated Mental Health Services for Older Adults: A Service Development Guide.,* Available from http://www.olderpeoplesmentalhealth.csip.org.uk/everybodys-business.html.

Cheng, J.S., Huang, W.F., Lin, K.M. and Shih, Y.T. (2008) Characteristics associated with benzodiazepine usage in elderly outpatients in Taiwan. *International Journal of Geriatric Psychiatry* 23(6): 618–24.

Chilvers, R., Harrison, G., Sipos, A. and Barley, M. (2002) Evidence into practice: application of psychological models of change in evidence based implementation. *British Journal of Psychiatry* 181(2): 99–101.

Clough, R., Hart, R., Nugent, M., Fox, D. and Watkins, C. (2004) *Older People and Alcohol*. Available from http://www.3sf.co.uk/download/SummaryFeb04.pdf.

Cowart, M. and Sutherland, M. (1998) Late life drinking among women. *Geriatric Nursing* 19(4): 214–19.

Currie, J. (2004) Manufacturing addiction: the over-prescription of benzodiazepines and sleeping pills to women in Canada. British Columbia Centre of Excellence for Women's Health Policy series. *Network Magazine of the Canadian Women's Health Network* 6/7(4/1): 16–19.

Davidson, R. (1992) Prochaska and DiClemente's model of change: a case study? *British Journal of Addiction* 87(6): 821–2.

Department of Health (2001) *National Service Framework for Older People*. Available from http://www.dh.gov.uk/en/Publicationsandstatistics/Publications/PublicationsPolicyAndGuidance/DH_4003066.

Department of Health (2005a) *Securing Better Mental Health for Older Adults*. Available from http://www.dh.gov.uk/en/Publicationsandstatistics/Publications/PublicationsPolicyAndGuidance/DH_4114989.

Department of Health (2005b) *Supporting People with Long Term Conditions*: *An NHS and Social Care Model to Support Local Innovation and Integration*. Available from http://www.dh.gov.uk/en/Publicationsandstatistics/Publications/PublicationsPolicyAndGuidance/DH_4100252.

Department of Health (2008) *National Service Framework for Older People and System Reform*. Available from http://www.dh.gov.uk/en/socialcare/Deliveringadultsocialcare/olderpeople/NSFforolderpeopleandsystemreform/index.htm.

Diabetes UK (2008) *Diabetes and Erectile Dysfunction*. Available from http://www.diabetes.co.uk/diabetes-erectile-dysfunction.html.

Duffin, C. (2008) Taking the risky out of frisky. *Nursing Older People* 20(5): 6–7.

Dyson, J. (2006) Alcohol misuse and older people. *Nursing Older People* 18(7): 32–5.

Ernst, E. and White, A. (2000) The BBC survey of complementary medicine use in the UK. *Complementary Therapies in Medicine* 8(1): 32–6.

Evandrou, M. (ed.) (1997) *Baby Boomers: Ageing in the 21st Century*. London: Age Concern England.

Evandrou, M. (2005) In Soule et al., *Focus on Older People: Health and Well Being*. Available from http://www.statistics.gov.uk/downloads/theme_compendia/foop05/Olderpeople2005.pdf.

Feldman, H.A., Goldstein, I., Hatzichristou, D.G., Krane, R.J., and McKinlay, J.B. (1994) Impotence and its medical and psychosocial correlates: results of the Massachusetts Male Aging Study. *Journal of Urology* 151(1): 54–61.

Finch, H. (1997) *Physical Activity at our Age*. London: Health Education Authority.

Finney, J., Moos, R. and Brennan, P. (1991) The Drinking Problems Index: a measure to assess alcohol related problems among older adults. *Journal of Substance Abuse* 3(4): 431–40.

French, J. and Blair-Stevens, C. (2005) *Social Marketing Pocket Guide*. London: National Consumer Council.

Gfroerer, J., Penne, M., Pemberton, M. and Folson, R. (2002) Substance abuse treatment need among older adults in 2020: the impact of the aging baby-boom cohort. *Drug and Alcohol Dependence* 69(2): 127–35.

Glanz, K., Rimer, B.K. and Lewis, F.M. (2002) *Health Behaviour and Health Education: Theory, Research and Practice*, 3rd edn. San Francisco: Jossey-Bass.

Glass, T., Mendes de Leon, C., Marottoli, R.A. and Berkman, L.F. (1999) Population based study of social and productive activities as predictors of survival among elderly Americans. *British Medical Journal* 319(7208): 478–83.

Goldberg, D., Bridges, K., Duncan-Jones, P. and Grayson, D. (1988) Detecting anxiety and depression in general medical settings. *British Medical Journal* 297(6693): 897–9.

Gossop, M. and Moos, R. (2008) Substance misuse among older adults: a neglected but treatable problem. *Addiction* 103(3): 347–8.

Hajat, S., Haines, A., Bulpitt, C. and Fletcher, A. (2004) Patterns and determinants of alcohol consumption in people aged 75 years and older: results from the MRC trial of assessments and management of older people in the community. *Age and Ageing* 33: 170–7.

Hansen-Kyle, L. (2005) A concept analysis of healthy ageing. *Nursing Forum* 40(2): 45–57.

Harwood, D.M., Hawton, K., Hope, T. and Jacoby, R. (2000) Suicide in older people: mode of death, demographic factors and medical contact before death. *International Journal of Geriatric Psychiatry* 15(8): 736–43.

Health Promotion Agency (2005) *Health Promotion Theories and Models*. Available from http://www.healthpromotionagency.org.uk/healthpromotion/health/section5.htm.

Heaphy, B., Yip, A. and Thompson, D. (2003) *Lesbian, Gay and Bisexual Lives Over 50: A Report on the Project 'The Social and Policy Implications of Non-heterosexual Ageing'*, Available from http://ess.ntu.ac.uk/heaphy/LGB50+.doc.

Heath, H. and Schofield, I. (1999) *Healthy Ageing, Nursing Older People*. London: Harcourt.

Help the Aged (2008) *All Change: Making Better Transport a Reality*. Available from http://www.helptheaged.org.uk/NR/rdonlyres/163AFCE7-A059-4B10-8973 DF000D1BABCC/0/ci_allchange_010607.pdf.

Hudson, A.J. and Moore, L.J. (2006) A new way of caring for older people in the community. *Nursing Standard* 40(26): 41–7.

Institute of Alcohol Studies (1999) *Alcohol and the Elderly Fact Sheet*. Available from www.ias.org.uk.

Jones, L. and Sidells M. (1997) *The Challenge of Promoting Health, Exploration and Action*. Basingstoke: Open University/Macmillan.

Katona, C.L.E. and Shankar, K.K. (1999) Depression in old age. *Reviews in Clinical Gerontology* 9 (4): 343–61.

Katz, J., Peberdy, A. and Douglas, J. (2000) *Promoting Health, Knowledge and Practice*, 2nd edn. Basingstoke: Open University/Macmillan.

Kellett, J. (1993) Sexuality in later life. *Reviews in Clinical Gerontology* 3: 309–14.

Kerr, S.M., Watson, H.E. and Tolson, D. (2002) Older people who smoke: why nurses should help them to stop. *British Journal of Nursing* 11(15): 1012–20.

Khan, N., Wilkinson, J. and Keeling, S. (2006) Reasons for changing alcohol use among older people in New Zealand. *Australasian Journal on Ageing* 25(2): 97–100.

Koloski, N., Smith, N., Pachana, N.A. and Dobson, A. (2008) Performance of the Goldberg Anxiety and Depression Scale in older women, *Age and Ageing*, 37: 464–7.

Kopera-Frye, K., Wiscott, R. and Sternss H.L. (1999) Can the drinking problem index provide valuable therapeutic information for recovering alcoholic adults? *Ageing and Mental Health* 3(3): 246–56.

Lach, W., Everard, K., Highstein, G. and Brownson, C. (2004) Application of the transtheoretical model to health education for older adults. *Health Promotion Practice* 5(1): 88–93.

Lakhani, N. (1997) Alcohol use amongst community dwelling elderly people: a review of the literature. *Journal of Advanced Nursing* 25(6): 1227–32.

Lambert, S., Granville, G., Lewis, J., Merrell, J. and Taylor, C. (2007) *'As soon as I get my Trainers on I Feel like Dancing': An Evaluation of Ageing Well in England and Wales.* Available from http://www.opanwales.org.uk/Portals/15/docs/AgeingWell.pdf.

Laurance, J. (2008) The new sexual revolution: over-70s are having more sex than ever – but more women than men are enjoying it. *Independent*, 9 July.

Lindau, S.T., Schumm, P., Laumann, E.O., Levinson, W., O'Muircheartaigh, C. and Waite, L. (2007) A study of sexuality and health in Older adults in the United States. *New England Journal of Medicine* 357(8): 762–74.

McGrath, A., Crome, P. and Crome, I.B. (2005) Substance misuse in the older population. *Postgraduate Medical Journal* 81(954): 228–31.

McVeigh, T. (2001) Over-65s ignore safe sex warnings. *Guardian*, 9 April.

Manthorpe, J. and Iliffe, S. (2005) Suicide among older people. *Nursing Older People* 17(10): 24–9.

Mayhew, L. (2005) Active ageing in the UK – issues, barriers, policy directions. *Innovation* 18(4): 455–77.

Mechanic, D. (1999) Issues in promoting health. *Social Science and Medicine* 48(6): 711–18.

Moos, R., Schutte, K., Brennan, P. and Moos, B. (2004) Ten year patterns of alcohol consumption and drinking problems among older women and men. *Addiction* 99(7): 829–38.

Moriarty, J. (2005) *Update for SCIE Best Practice Guide on Assessing the Mental Health Needs of Older People.* Available from http://www.scie.org.uk/publications/practiceguides/practiceguide02/files/research.pdf.

Mottram, P., Wilson, K. and Strobl, J. (2006) Antidepressants for depressed elderly. *Cochrane Database of Systematic Reviews.* Available from http://www.cochrane.org/reviews/.

Naik, P. and Jones, R.G. (1994) Alcohol histories taken from elderly people on admission. *British Medical Journal* 308: 248.

National Cancer Institute (2005) *Theory at a Glance: A Guide for Health Promotion Practice.* Available from, http://www.nci.nih.gov/pdf/481f5d53-63df-41bc-bfaf-5aa48ee1da4d/TAAG3.pdf.

National Institute for Health and Clinical Excellence (2008) *Promoting Mental Well Being in Older People.* Available from http://www.nice.org.uk/nicemedia/pdf/MentalHealth_draftscope.pdf.

National Institute for Mental Health in England (2005) *Making it Possible: Improving Mental Health and Well-being in England.* London: NIMHE.

National Social Marketing Centre (2006) *It's our Health: Realising the Potential for Effective Social Marketing.* Available from http://www.nsms.org.uk/images/CoreFiles/Recognising_It_When_You_See_ItNSMS.doc.

Nigg, C., Burbank, P., Padula, C. et al. (1999) Stages of change across ten health risk behaviours for older adults. *Gerontologist* 39(4): 473–82.

O'Connell, H., Chin, A., Cunningham, C. and Lawlor, B. (2003) Alcohol use disorders in elderly people – redefining an age old problem in old age. *British Medical Journal* 327(7416): 664–7.

Organisation for Economic Cooperation and Development (1998) *Maintaining Prosperity in an Ageing Society: Background Report.* Available from http://www.oecd.org/dataoecd/21/10/2430300.pdf.

Osborn, D.P.J., Fletcher, A.E., Smeeth, L. et al. (2003) Factors associated with depression in a representative sample of 14 217 people aged 75 and over in the United Kingdom: results from the MRC trial of assessment and management of older people in the community. *International Journal of Geriatric Psychiatry* 18(7): 623–30.

Parry, O., Thomson, C. and Fowkes, G. (2002) Cultural context, older age and smoking in Scotland: qualitative interviews with older smokers with arterial disease. *Health Promotion International* 17(4): 309–15.

Persson, G. (1980) Sexuality in a 70 year old urban population. *Journal of Psychosomatic Research* 24: 335–42.

Phillips, P. and Katz, A. (2001) Substance misuse in older adults: an emerging policy priority. *NT Research* 6(6): 898–905.

Philp, I. (2002) Developing a National Service Framework for Older People. *Journal of Epidemiology and Community Health* 56(11): 841–2.

Philp, I. (2004) *Better Health in Old Age: Resource Document.* Available from http://www.dh.gov.uk/en/Publicationsandstatistics/Publications/PublicationsPolicyAndGuidance/DH_4092840.

Philpot, M., Pearson, N., Petratou, V., Dayanandan, R., Silverman, M. and Marshall, J. (2003) Screening for problem drinking in older people referred to a mental health service: a comparison of CAGE and AUDIT. *Ageing and Mental Health* 7(3): 171–5.

Prochaska, J. and DiClemente, C. (1983) Stages and processes of self-change of smoking: toward an integrative model of change. *Journal of Consulting and Clinical Psychology* 51(3): 390–5.

Prochaska, J., Norcross, J. and DiClemente, C. (2006) *Changing for Good.* Available from http://www.positiveworkplace.com.

Rai, D.K. and Finch, H. (1997) *Physical Activity from our Point of View*. London: Health Education Authority.

Redfern, S. and Ross, F. (eds.) (2006) *Nursing Older People*: London: Churchill Livingstone.

Reicherter, E. and Greene, R. (2005) Wellness and health promotion: educational applications for older adults in the community, *Topics in Geriatric Rehabilitation* 21(4): 295–303.

Resnik, B. (2003) Health promotion practices of older adults: model testing. *Public Health Nursing* 20(1): 2–12.

Rogstad, K. and Bignell, C. (1991) Age is no bar to sexually acquired infection. *Age and Ageing* 20(5): 377–8.

Ross, R.K., Bernstein, L., Trent, L., Henderson, B.E. and Paganini-Hill, A. (1990) A prospective study of risk factors for traumatic death in the retirement community. *Preventive Medicine* 19(3): 323–34.

Sabin, E. (1993) Social relationships and mortality among the elderly. *Journal of Applied Gerontology* 12(1): 44–60.

Seedhouse, D. (1995) *Health the Foundations of Achievement*. Chichester: John Wiley and Sons.

Seniors Network (2008) *Myths of Ageing*. Available from http://www.seniorsnetwork.co.uk/grandparents/mythsofaging.htm.

Shah, A. and Fountain, J. (2008) Illicit drug use and problematic use in the elderly: is there a case for concern? *International Psychogeriatrics* (April 17): 1–9.

Soule, A., Babb, P., Evandrou, M., Balchin, S. and Zealey, L. (2005) Focus on older people, National Statistics Office and Department for work and pensions, HMSO: London, available from http://www.statistics.gov.uk/downloads/theme_compendia/foop05/Olderpeople2005.pdf.

Speller, V., Learmonth, A. and Harrison, D. (1998) The search for evidence of effective health promotion. *British Medical Journal* 316(7132): 361–3.

Strachan, I. (2001) Medicines and older people: a nurses' guide to administration. *British Journal of Community Nursing* 6(6): 296–301.

Swedish National Institute of Health (2007) *Healthy Ageing – a Challenge for Europe*. Available from http://www.healthyageing.nu/templates/page.aspx?id=1321.

Szasz, G. (1983) Sexual incidents in an extended care unit for aged men. *Journal of the American Geriatrics Society* 31(7): 407–411.

Todd, C. and Skelton, D. (2004) *What are the Main Risk Factors for Falls Among Older People and What Are the Most Effective Interventions to Prevent these Falls?* Health Evidence Network report. Available from http://www.euro.who.int/document/E82552.pdf.

University of Twente (2004) *Health Belief Model*. Available from http://www.tcw.utwente.nl.

Victor, C. (2000) *Promoting the Health of Older People, Setting a Research Agenda*. London: Health Development Agency.

Vincent, C., Ridell, J. and Shmueli, A. (2000) *Sexuality and Older Women – Setting the Scene*. London: Tavistock Marital Studies Institute.

Weinstein, N. (1988) The precaution adoption process. *Health Psychology* 7(4): 355–86.

Wellman, B., Kelner, M. and Wigdor, B. (2001) Older adults' use of medical and alternative care. *Journal of Applied Gerontology* 20(1): 3–23.

Whelan, G. (2003) Alcohol: a much neglected risk factor in elderly mental disorders. *Current Opinion in Psychiatry* 16(6): 609–14.

White, I. (2001) Facilitating sexual expression: challenges for current practice. In H. Heath and I. White (eds.) *Challenging Sexuality in Health Care*. Oxford: Blackwell Science.

Whitehead, D. (2001) Health education, behavioural change and social psychology: nursing's contribution to health promotion? *Journal of Advanced Nursing* 34(6): 822–32.

Whitehead, D. (2004) Health promotion and health education: advancing the concepts. *Journal of Advanced Nursing* 47(3): 311–20.

World Health Organization (1990) *International Classification of Disease Revision 10*. Available from http://www.who.int/classifications/icd/en/.

World Health Organization (2006) *Health Promotion and Education*. Available from http://www.searo.who.int/en/Section1174/Section1458.htm.

World Health Organization (2008) *What is "Active Ageing"?* Available from http://www.who.int/ageing/active_ageing/en/print.html.

Wright, L. and Bramwell, R. (2001) A qualitative study of older people's perceptions of skin cancer. *Health Education Journal* 60(3): 256–64.

Young, K. (1996) Health, health promotion and the elderly. *Journal of Clinical Nursing* 5(4): 241–8.

Zollman, C. and Vickers, A. (1999) The ABC of complementary medicine: what is complementary medicine? *British Medical Journal* 319(7211): 693–6.

Useful websites

Alcohol Concern: http://www.alcoholconcern.org.uk

Alcoholics Anonymous: http://www.alcoholics-anonymous.org.uk

Council for Information on Tranquillisers and Antidepressants: http://www.citawithdrawal.org.uk/index.html

Cruse Bereavement Care: http://www.crusebereavementcare.org.uk/

Down your Drink: https://www.downyourdrink.org.uk/index.jsp

Dry Out Now: http://www.dryoutnow.com

Extend: http://www.extend.org.uk/

Geriatric Depression Scale: http://www.patient.co.uk/showdoc/40002438/

Help the Aged: http://www.helptheaged.org.uk

National Coalition for Active Ageing: http://www.laterlifetraining.co.uk/documents/NCCAFinal.pdf

Samaritans: http://www.samaritans.org/

Survivors of Bereavement by Suicide: http://www.uk-sobs.org.uk/

Women's Health Concern: www.womens-health-concern.org

Chapter 5

Older people with learning disabilities

Kim Scarborough

Introduction

In every 1000 people in the UK, three or four will have a severe learning disability and 25–30 will have a mild learning disability (Emerson et al. 2001), indicating there are up to 2 million people with learning disabilities in the UK. Numbers are increasing, and increased longevity is resulting in this section of society experiencing age-related illnesses (Jancar 1998). Although they have an ordinary life expectancy, these citizens are more likely to die before their non-disabled peers and four times more likely to die of a preventable cause (Hollins et al. 1998). In addition, people with learning disabilities develop age-related health problems earlier than the general population (Department of Health [DH] 2001a, 2001b). This chapter will explore the healthcare and community issues of ageing for people who have a learning disability.

Defining learning disability

People who have a learning disability are not a homogenous group. The World Health Organization (1996) uses the term 'mental retardation' and states that having an IQ below 70 and difficulties in social functioning that occurred before the age of 18 indicates a learning disability. UK definitions include the above, referring to learning disabilities being a life-long condition, with the existence of global difficulties with intellectual functioning and adaptive behaviours resulting in a need for support throughout their lives (Emerson et al. 2001). The self-advocacy organisation

People First regard the term 'mental retardation' as pejorative owing to the abusive use of the words that have developed in our culture. It is not a term that health practitioners use; however, when searching the literature, it is advisable to use the World Health Organization terminology as a key word to ensure access to international research papers. Preferred terms are 'learning disability', 'learning difficulty' and 'intellectual impairment'. The term 'learning disability' will be used throughout this chapter because it is the language used in recent UK health legislation. The degree of disability is recorded as mild, moderate, severe or profound.

Individuals with *mild learning disabilities* will be fairly independent, possibly with their own home, job and intimate relationships. Individuals may experience difficulties with literacy and numeracy and take longer to learn new skills than their non-disabled peers. Although individuals often have a wide vocabulary, it can be difficult for them to understand the complexities of language, resulting in health professionals thinking that the person has a better understanding of information than they actually have.

Individuals with *moderate learning disabilities* require higher levels of support to live independently and may have jobs and intimate relationships. Numeracy and literacy skills will be poor, and learning new skills will take time and practice. Communication skills are reduced, but the use of accessible language and information will ensure that people are as fully involved as possible in decisions about their health.

Individuals with *severe learning disabilities* will have limited independent living skills and require daily support. Communication skills will be limited, and the use of augmentative and alternative communication (AAC) tools will enhance understanding. People will be able to make choices, and care should be taken to ensure that their choices are understood. However, their capacity to give consent may need to be assessed, and therefore it should not be assumed that the person is unable to give consent in some areas of his or her life. Individuals are more likely to have additional health needs, including epilepsy and sensory impairments.

Individuals with *profound and multiple learning disabilities* (PMLD) will have very limited or no self-care skills and require high levels of support throughout the day and possibly night. They experience considerable communication difficulties, and the use of AACs may aid their understanding. Often, individuals use idiosyncratic communication that carers are best placed to interpret. The individual is more likely to have severe mobility, neurological and health problems (MENCAP 2007b).

Whatever the degree of disability, the health practitioner must ensure that the individual is at the centre of health assessments and interventions, and not speak only to the carer, but ensure things are explained to individuals in ways to promote their understanding and promote control of their own health.

Recent policy and people with learning disabilities

Historically, people with learning disabilities have received poor education, social and healthcare. Older people may have received segregated education, and many were cared for in institutions until the development of community care services in the 1980s. Those who stayed at home to be cared for by family members had limited contact with their communities. This segregation resulted in the health needs of people with learning disabilities being largely unmet (Disability Rights Commission [DRC] 2006). Health professionals have not developed the skills and knowledge needed to provide good quality healthcare (DH 2001a), as demonstrated in high-profile reports by MENCAP such as *Treat Me Right* (2003a) and *Death by Indifference* (2007a).

Valuing People (DH 2001a) is the first government paper in England on learning disabilities in 30 years. It has consolidated research, human rights issues and the experiences of people with learning disabilities and their families into a strategy document that is helping to give a focus for service improvements. The paper states that person-centred plans should be developed for older people with learning disabilities from the age of 50 to ensure appropriate support as they age. In addition, the *National Service Framework for Older People* (DH 2001b) and recent papers such as *Our Health, Our Care, Our Say* (DH 2006) discuss health education, health choices and equitable healthcare for all. Such papers apply to all citizens, including those who have learning disabilities.

Impact of having a learning disability

Knowing that a person has a learning disability says very little about them or how to meet their needs. As with anyone, health professionals need to get to know the individual and not make assumptions based on labels and diagnoses. This does not mean that if a cause of a person's learning disability is known, one should ignore it. A specific diagnosis such as Down's syndrome might indicate a significantly higher risk of some medical conditions, and understanding these risks can be helpful when supporting an older individual to be healthy.

Another consequence of having a learning disability is that people age more quickly, with age-related illness starting as early as 50 years of age

(Hatzidimitriadou and Milne 2005). In some people, for example those with Downs syndrome or PMLD, this can occur even earlier, with higher risks of premature death. Also, age-related sight impairment can occur 10 years earlier than in the general population (Starling et al. 2006). Scope (2007) report how people with cerebral palsy can experience physical deterioration due to the long-term effects of living with impairments, experiencing new or increased pain and joint, muscle and continence problems. It is fundamental that health changes are identified early and managed to maximise health and maintain functioning levels into old age.

The main cause of death in people with learning disabilities is respiratory disease, followed by heart disease (Hollins et al. 1998); death from cancer is on the increase (Duff et al. 2001). Contributing lifestyle factors could be that these citizens have difficulty interpreting public health messages about keeping healthy, are more likely to be under or overweight than the general population, and may be less likely to eat a balanced diet (Robertson et al. 2000a). Also, individuals are less able to report ill-health, and do not receive health checks at which health problems can be detected early, including reduced attendance for screening for breast, cervical or testicular cancers (Djuretic et al. 1999).

Being older with learning disabilities can mean that people lose contact with family and networks including long-term paid carers (Hatzidimitriadou and Milne 2005). Bland et al. (2003) reported that older people who lived in residential care homes had very limited contact with family members. This can impact on mental and physical health, meaning that meeting the social and relationship needs of people with learning disabilities is important for their well-being.

Communicating with older people with learning disabilities

A common feature of people with learning disabilities is communication difficulties, often exacerbated during illness because of anxiety, pain and previous experiences of healthcare. An individual might need support from a carer who can interpret changes in behaviour and non-verbal communication to indicate illness. But carers can misinterpret or be unaware of such changes, especially if symptoms are pain free (DH 1998). Health professionals need to ensure that carers are fully aware of potential signs and symptoms. Keeping behaviour, signs and symptoms diaries are useful for recording possible indicators of health changes or drug side-effects, and can provide a medium for dialogue between people with learning disabilities, carers and health professionals. It is essential that if a person has behaviour changes, possible physical causes are explored and such changes are not misinterpreted as challenging behaviour.

> **Reflection points**
>
> • Reflect upon the five principles of the *Human Rights in Healthcare – a Framework for Local Action* (DH 2007a), identified in Chapter 3, and consider how these can be applied to the care of people with learning disabilities.

Since 1983, the problems with identifying and self-reporting ill-health have been documented (Bland et al. 2003). People with learning disabilities might lack the vocabulary to discuss health issues, or they may think their symptoms are an accepted part of ageing. People may have had limited health education and be unaware of the significance of particular signs and symptoms. Some individuals may have a reasonable health vocabulary but limited understanding of the words they use and be acquiescent; resulting in people leaving a consultation misunderstanding what has been said. It is good practice to give people with learning disabilities double appointments, allowing adequate time to check understanding and reinforce significant points, as well as to give them accessible information to take away and review.

Good communication systems and skills are essential in reducing health inequalities. However, as the label 'learning disability' is applied to a broad spectrum of people, such systems and skills have to be person centred. Good practice is to have a communication plan that is easy to read with key points unambiguously recorded and the document read before an appointment. Important things to include are communication strategies – any routines that might help gain the person's attention or trust, and individuals' reactions to common health interventions such as taking blood. Examples of communication and admission frameworks are the *Traffic Light Assessment* (Gloucestershire Partnership NHS Trust 2005) and *All About Me* (Rose 2006), available from *Access to Acute Care: Supporting People with a Learning Disability on Admission to Hospital* (Access to Acute 2007) on the National Network for Learning Disability Nurses website (see Useful websites at the end of the chapter).

Strategies for maximising communication are to use simple words and no health jargon, and to give one instruction at a time, for example, 'Sit down,' (wait), 'Take off your shoes' (wait), 'Show me your foot.' If given as one continuous instruction, people may forget the sequence and get confused, anxious or angry. It is also important that sentences are short, with one topic to enhance understanding. It is important to give people time to process what has been said, and to reply. Avoid negatives as they are difficult to understand. For example say, 'Please keep your foot still,' and not 'I'd rather you did not move your foot.' The latter might make people move their foot more as they have only processed the last three words. Finally, time spent checking that the person understands and identifying how to give information for further review is important because people usually have poor memories and need to go over information at their own pace.

People with autism will have difficulties using ordinary communication styles and systems. As Plimley (2007: 208) writes, 'variety is not the spice of life', and people with autism need familiarity, consistency and predictability, especially at a time when ill-health causes them stress. Strategies to help set these parameters are about advanced planning. Having opportunities, when well, to familiarise themselves with staff, medical facilities, equipment and procedures can reduce anxiety. In addition, having an agreed plan for what will happen should an individual become ill can help future contact be more successful. The time to work with carers to prepare an access plan that stipulates double appointments, times of the day when the person is most likely to cope with an appointment, reactions to waiting, and meeting any sensory needs can reduce anxiety and maximise the potential for a successful environment in which to discuss health concerns. Sensory differences are common for people with autism, and knowing in advance that a person might be wearing earphones because they experience pain with some noises or that they cannot tolerate specific fabrics or touch (Plimley 2007) can ensure the health practitioner maintains an environment conducive to a positive outcome.

AAC tools are used by some people with learning disabilities. Although not expecting expertise from the health practitioner, a basic understanding of AACs is useful on their part. Where people use AACs, it is helpful for the health practitioner to ask the carer how to use them so that they can interact with the patient. AACs are varied and include:

- TEACHH: a communication tool often used with people who have autism
- Makaton symbols: represent key words and concepts
- Makaton and e-sign: key word sign languages. Learning a few signs might help build rapport
- Objects of reference: real or representational objects used to indicate choices and needs
- Images: line drawings or photographs that can be shown or pointed at
- Communication passports: a person-centred resource used by people with severe and profound learning disabilities.

Total Communication (Jones 2001) is where a person uses a mixture of AACs to enhance effective two-way communication. It is good practice to continue using verbal language, gesture and physical cues alongside any AACs.

Paper-based information for health education is widely used with the general public, but can be inaccessible to and not meet the needs of people with learning disabilities. Basic rules for making accessible health resources are to use easy words, pictures directly related to the topic, and a good layout with lots of white space and a minimum of a 16-point font. It is advisable to use sentence case because capitals are more difficult to read, and to use an Arial or Comic Sans typeface, which does not have serifs. To develop these skills, it is advisable to read and evaluate good accessible information; such material can be found on the DH website and is available from the British Institute of Learning Disabilities.

Individual coaching and mentoring for good health is being developed with the introduction of health trainers. Health trainers are people from communities where health inequalities exist (DH 2005). In Bristol and South Gloucestershire, people with learning disabilities are becoming health trainers (Scarborough 2008). For older people with learning disabilities who need support to understand healthy lifestyles, coaching relationships could be of benefit in helping them to understand, gain motivation and take control of their own health.

Vulnerability

People with learning disability are a marginalised group, and older people generally are not valued by society. So to be older and have a learning disability presents the individual with double discrimination and its ensuing vulnerabilities (Respond 2007). One major difference for older people with learning disabilities is that they are much less likely to have adult children who can 'keep an eye' on them or social networks that can provide support (Respond 2007). Older people with learning disabilities are more likely to live with non-related adults, which is linked to a higher risk of abuse. They are also less likely to be able to comprehend home and personal safety messages that their non-disabled peers receive and understand. Recent reports of mistreatment indicate that having live-in staff does not necessarily decrease how vulnerable a person is to abuse (Commission for Social Care Inspection 2006). Visiting health professionals are well placed to report suspected abuse. In addition, there is a long history of bullying and victimisation of people with learning disabilities, with individuals being targeted by non-disabled people within their communities (Whittell and Ramcharan 2000). These vulnerabilities need careful consideration and management if physical and mental health is to be maximised.

Principles underpinning services for people with learning disabilities

The principles stated in *Valuing People* (DH 2001a) underpin health and social care services for people with learning disabilities. These are inclusion, rights, choice and control. *Inclusion* means that people are active members of their community, with valued roles, personal contacts and a sense of belonging. People are able to access mainstream services and specialist services as indicated by their individual needs. *Rights* are highlighted because people with learning disabilities have a history of their rights being subjugated, and people have struggled to be recognised as having equal rights to their non-disabled peers. This includes the right to equality of healthcare. *Choice* and *control* are key themes driving change, for example accessible information, sufficient time, being listened to and having choices respected. Forbat (2006: 258) writes how these four principles 'have particular resonance' for older people with learning disabilities. She indicates this is due to older people with learning disabilities experiencing less inclusion, rights, control and choices.

Community services and support systems for older people with learning disabilities

There is a range of service options for older people with learning disabilities, but there are also gaps in knowledge and services. Plimley (2007) identified the lack of research into meeting the needs of older people with autism, stating that the majority of good practice developments focus on younger people. Good practice recommendations are therefore extrapolated for this group. Alongside this dearth of knowledge related to some groups, there are wide knowledge bases being developed about supporting people with Down's syndrome as they age.

Living in the family home

The majority of people with learning disabilities, including many older people, live with a family member (Thompson 2002), and parents often want to provide care for as long as possible (Hatzidimitriadou and Milne 2005). Problems can occur when people are not known to services, and when their carer dies they lose not only a parent, but also their home and neighbours when they are placed in a care setting. Bland et al. (2003) state how older people with learning disabilities living with family carers have not been a priority group, with Thompson (2002) adding that specialist learning disabilities services are themselves ageist, abdicating responsibility when an older person needs support for the first time. The role of people with learning disabilities as carer to an elderly parent is rarely recognised, but a visiting health professional might identify this interdependence. Where any of these issues are recognised, the involvement of specialist services to instigate planning for the future should be discussed with the family.

Respite care

Respite care can be provided at home or through specialist respite service providers. Uptake of hospice services is generally low. Families can have difficulties accessing respite care, causing high levels of stress (MENCAP 2003b).

Independent living

Increasingly, people with learning disabilities live independently in their own home. They may have no contact with specialist learning disabilities services, and as their support networks age, they may become isolated (Hatzidimitriadou and Milne 2005). People may have had to fight for their right to live independently and not want to jeopardise their living arrangements by asking for extra support.

Specialist residential and nursing homes for people with learning disabilities

Many people live in specialist residential homes, which can be ordinary houses or purpose-built homes. Staff may have little understanding of ageing or health and need education to provide continuing care. Specialist nursing homes tend to cater for people who have high health needs. These tend to be people with PMLD and life-limiting conditions so there is usually a younger population.

Residential communities

These are campus-style services with a variety of homes in one location owned by one service provider. These are not the same as the institutions managed by the National Health Service (NHS), which are all but closed. These private and voluntary organisations offer choice to families and people with learning disabilities about the type of services they wish to receive.

Residential and nursing homes for older people

With the move towards inclusion, older people with learning disabilities are using mainstream older people's services. Although this can be successful and is viewed as a positive step to inclusion, authors such as Thompson (2002) point out that the philosophies and funding levels between learning disabilities and older persons' services are different. The Foundation for People with Learning Disabilities (FPLD; 2001) identified a skills and knowledge gap related to learning disabilities in the staff of older people's services, resulting in reduced opportunities for activities, stimulation and community-based activities, and reduced contact with family and friends. Another concern was that people with learning disabilities living in older people's services were significantly younger than other service users. *Valuing People* (DH 2001a) states that active older people with learning disabilities should not be placed in older people's services where residents are older, frailer and have higher health needs. Fit older people with learning disabilities do not have the same needs as other residents, resulting in high levels of unmet need.

Day care, work and occupation

Older people with learning disabilities are less likely to have had similar experiences of employment to their non-disabled peers. Many will have received day care in specialist units. However, since the publication of *Valuing People* (DH 2001a), this is changing, with more people working. Where people have not been part of the workforce, concepts such as retirement may not be understood. However, as day services are modernised and directed towards working-age adults, older people can have an unexpected enforced retirement. There are few day or leisure services specifically for older people with learning disabilities where friendships can be maintained and activities shared. Bigby (2005) suggests this needs to change, with older people with learning disabilities having the choice to access activities alongside younger people with learning disabilities, to attend older people clubs or to use specialist clubs for older people with learning disabilities. Limited social skills and reduced day occupation can result in extreme isolation.

Impact of ageing on where an older person with learning disability lives

As people with learning disability age, the appropriateness of their housing may become an issue for them or those they live with. Wilkinson et al. (2004) discuss three models of care: ageing in place, in-place progression and referral out.

Ageing in place

Ageing in place is where the older person with learning disabilities is supported to remain in his or her present accommodation, possibly requiring adaptation of the building or the acquisition of aids. Wilkinson et al. (2004) consider this to be the preferred model. Education and support for the individual is needed as many have insight into the negative impact that their ageing has on co-residents; however, this is not always offered (Forbat and Wilkinson 2008). Also, education for both family and paid carers helps ageing in place to be successful. Forbat and Wilkinson (2008) noted that where there are co-residents, their education about ageing and having opportunities to discuss problems experienced with an ageing co-resident can enhance the lives of all parties. Ageing in place support for families might mean respite care.

In-place progression

In-place progression is where specialist residential service providers for people with learning disabilities manage a range of homes. The same service provider continues to provide care but in another part of their organisation. Wilkinson et al. (2004) felt this results in the older person receiving continuity of care and greater opportunities to maintain relationships. In-place progression when the person lives at home may mean an existing respite or day services provider who knows the person well extending their service to offer additional residential care.

Referral out

Referral out is when a family or service is no longer able to meet the older person's needs and they are referred to alternative services, usually services for older people. Although staff in older people's services will have expertise in meeting their client's needs, they may have limited experience in meeting the needs of an older person with learning disabilities (Wilkinson et al. 2004). Diagnostic overshadowing can occur when staff misjudge behaviour changes. Where input from specialist learning disability services is requested, it is often to advise on the management of challenging behaviours that are misunderstood as related to learning disability when they are actually ill-health-related communication strategies (Hemmings and Greig 2007).

Health services and older people with learning disabilities

Although people with a learning disability are at higher risks of developing age-related health problems (DH 2001a, Kerr et al. 2003), it is worth stating that ill-health in old age is not a given. Health education and health checks can have a positive effect on older people with learning disabilities, helping them maintain good health for as long as possible. *Valuing People* (DH 2001a) states that people with a learning disability have an entitlement to quality healthcare that meets their individual needs. This relates to both primary and specialist healthcare. The *National Service Framework for Older People* (DH 2001b) concurs and directs for a needs-led service. The services discussed below must communicate effectively and plan in partnership so people can be fully supported.

Primary care

Bland et al. (2003) confirmed that the key health professionals for older people with learning disabilities are the GP and the primary care community nurses. Although people were generally satisfied with their healthcare, Bland discovered significant failings in health screening and annual health checks. Annual health checks are now part of primary care contracts, as outlined in the *Primary Care Service Framework,* with health action plans and health promotion as key aims (DH 2007b). There are significant barriers to accessing health screening, including assumptions about the ability of people to cooperate with and understand screening, poor communication systems, a lack of accessible health information, and health staff unskilled in communicating with, and gaining consent from, people with learning disabilities. These barriers result in health inequalities and, for some people, late diagnosis and premature death from treatable illnesses (MENCAP 2003a, 2007a; DRC 2006).

Specialist community learning disability teams

Community learning disability teams (CLDTs) are teams who specialise in the health and well-being of people with learning disabilities. Teams consist of health and social care professionals, with core team members being the learning disability nurse, occupational therapist, physiothera-pist, psychologist, psychiatrist, speech and language therapist, social worker and support staff. Teams can help generic health and social care staff develop a better understanding of the complexity of supporting someone who has a learning disability. As well as the support and educa-tion of others, they offer targeted assessment, interventions and person-centred care plans for people with learning disabilities. GPs should have the contact information for the local CLDT and can make referrals. Many CLDTs have accessible health resources or information about where resources can be found.

Mental health services

People with learning disabilities also have a higher risk of experienc-ing mental ill-health but experience poor mental healthcare provision (Hassiotis et al. 2000); however, *Valuing People* (DH 2001a) has chal-lenged services to participate in joint planning of care to enable equal access to mainstream services.

Health of older people with learning disabilities

Despite the fact that it has been known for many years that people with learning disabilities have higher risks of developing health problems and experience more health conditions, they continue to experience poor healthcare provision and as a result live with unmet health needs (DH 1998, 2001a; MENCAP 2003a, 2007a; DRC 2006). This results in four times as many people with learning disabilities dying from a treatable illness compared with the general public (DRC 2006). MENCAP pro-duced a report called *Death by Indifference* that presents evidence of poor quality treatment in the NHS resulting in possible preventable deaths. Identifying the causes of poor health is complex; undoubtedly some people are predisposed to certain health conditions, but unhealthy lifestyles, poor health education, poverty, mental ill-health and inaccessible health services conspire with low expectations and negative attitudes to result in today's health inequalities (Scenario 5.1).

Scenario 5.1: Len's health experiences

Len is 59 years old and lives at home with his 64-year-old sister Jean. He is fun to be with, enjoys shopping, loves watching TV and works with Jean as a secret shopper, letting auditors know if shop assistants provide good customer service. Len has severe learning disabilities and communication difficulties so he uses a computer to help him talk to other people. He has epilepsy, uses a wheelchair, cannot stand up and often has problems with his bowels. However, Jean considers him to be generally healthy and happy.

A few weeks ago, however, Jean noticed that he was not eating very much. He appeared to be constipated, and despite giving him his usual oral medication, he still did not defaecate. Getting to an appointment at the surgery was always a problem, and Len's sister did not want to waste people's time so, as on previous occasions, she contacted the surgery and asked for a prescription for suppositories. The practice nurse had a brief conversation with her confirming 'the usual' and sorted out a prescription. Jean later administered the suppository and Len did have a small, very watery bowel movement.

However, he continued to eat little and started to show what Jean reported as signs of distress. She took him to an appointment at the surgery. At the surgery, there were lots of people waiting and a temporary GP on duty. Len had an allotted single appointment, and after waiting for nearly 45 minutes was rather uncooperative with the GP. There was nothing written on the notes about Len's communication device so the GP talked to Jean, seeming to ignore Len. No hoist was available to help Len onto the examination table, so the GP did a brief examination of Len's tummy while he was in his wheelchair – it was very brief because Len was unhappy and tried to bite the GP. The GP agreed it was severe constipation and prescribed an enema, which Jean gave when they got home, to some effect.

Len continued not to eat and started to refuse drinks, he showed signs of distress, and Jean thought he was in pain. This had now been a problem for nearly 3 weeks and Len was losing weight. Jean phoned the surgery and tried to get an appointment for Len to see his own GP but it was not possible, so she settled for an appointment with another temporary GP. After another 50 minutes' wait and a cursory examination with no attempt to communicate directly with Len, the GP sent Len for an X-ray that revealed a bowel blockage. Len was admitted to hospital for medical intervention. During his time, there his antiepileptic medication was not given for 24 hours, resulting in Len having increased seizures. He had a nasogastric tube and a colostomy on discharge. Jean was taught how to care for these and Len was sent home. The community team were contacted and arrangements made for them to support Len and Jean in caring for the nasogastric tube and colostomy.

Reflection points

- What were the barriers experienced by Len and Jean?
- What could the receptionist do during booking and while Len was waiting to see the doctor?
- How might communication with Len be improved?
- What might a practice nurse do with Len and Jean before Len became ill again to enable effective future consultations?
- How might the community team caring for Len when he is discharged home ensure the best possible outcomes for Len and his family?
- How might the health centre staff improve the support for Len and Jean next time he becomes ill?

Healthcare practitioners have a responsibility to provide good healthcare for people with learning disabilities, but they may need training to do this. Self-advocacy organisations such as People First provide training to help consider staff's values and raise awareness of the needs of people with learning disabilities. Health professionals usually only meet people with learning disabilities when the individuals are ill and possibly stressed, so having an opportunity to listen to people in a learning environment can allow staff to ask questions and consider their practice. These encounters give health professionals an opportunity to discuss issues of access, how services are perceived and how they might improve their provision.

Specific health issues for people with learning disabilities

Mental health

People with learning disabilities have a higher risk of developing mental illness than the general population, with prevalence rates of 40–50%; there is a three times higher risk of schizophrenia, and older people with learning disabilities have a particularly higher risk of depression and anxiety (Collacott et al. 1998; Doody et al. 1998; Bland et al. 2003; Smiley 2005; Cooper et al. 2007). Xenitidis et al. (2003) found that many people who had learning disabilities and mental health problems felt that non-learning-disability mental health workers failed to recognise when a mental illness was present and, if a diagnosis was made, their treatment was not always comparable to that given to non-disabled patients. It was suggested by Hemmings and Greig (2007) that some older people with learning disabilities and mental health problems required healthcare specialising in the diagnosis and treatment of complex mental illness present in people with learning disability. However, this can prove difficult as mental health and learning disability services do not always have good lines of communication (Hassiotis et al. 2000), therefore reducing the opportunities for partnership working. The prevention of mental illness is paramount, and as such people's emotional and psychological, as well as physical, needs have to be met. This includes providing social interactions (Bland et al. 2003).

Older people with learning disabilities may experience multiple losses, and as they are highly susceptible to stress when bereaved, support is essential (Respond 2007). Although people experience stress following bereavement, they receive minimal support and, anecdotally, non-learning-disability trained health staff feel unskilled in helping an individual during bereavement. There are, however, steps that professionals can take. Read and Elliot (2007) present a bereavement support model stating that everyone will eventually experience bereavement, but for many people with learning disability, grief is unrecognised, not acknowledged or not accepted, individuals being excluded from participating in cultural rituals surrounding death, which results in their disenfranchisement. Read and Elliot refer to the 'continuum of bereavement support' (p. 171) as being education, participation, facilitation and intervention. This involves education about the life-cycle where death is normal, the process of dying, the language of death and dying and reactions to death, alongside participating in death rituals, for example visiting people who are dying, involvement in funerals and facilitating space to explore feelings. Taking opportunities as they arise can help facilitate this, for example discussing story lines in TV soap operas, and also using bereavement resources developed for people with learning disabilities by organisations such as Bereavement and Learning Disability.

Physical health

Older people with learning disabilities are at higher risk of some health conditions partly due to the link between some syndromes and medical conditions. Also, the long-term use of medication such antiepilepsy drugs, the higher risk of physical impairment and previously discussed health inequalities are all contributing factors. Areas to consider when providing healthcare for those at higher risk include the following.

Dementia

There is a higher risk of dementia for people with learning disabilities (Cooper 1997), especially those with Down's syndrome, with an early onset from 40 years of age and a more rapid progression of the disease once diagnosed (Holland et al. 1998). There are specific assessment tools for screening this population that are more sensitive to their needs; these are the Dementia Questionnaire for Mentally Retarded Persons and the Adaptive Behaviour Scale – Residential and Community (Strydom and Hassiotis 2003). With the significant risk for people with learning disabilities to develop dementia, baseline assessments against which future assessments can be measured is best practice, with a recommendation for these to happen at age 40 for people with Down's syndrome, and at 50 for all people with learning disabilities (Kirk et al. 2006).

Cancer

Although a lower incidence of cancer in people with learning disabilities was reported in the 1980–90s, recent research with this client group (Hermon et al. 2001; Sullivan et al. 2005) has identified a higher risk specifically of gastrointestinal cancer, leukaemia and brain cancers in men, and leukaemia, uterine and colon cancers in women, with upward trends in age-related cancers. They also reported late diagnosis, when cancer is less treatable. Good practice is to ensure that people receive accessible invitations and advice about screening and, if needed, are reminded to attend on the day of the appointment. Time spent explaining the procedure is important, with preparatory visits helping to reduce anxiety. Accessible resources have been written by Books Beyond Words, including *Looking after my Breasts* and *Looking after my Balls*, and CHANGE is currently writing a series about a range of cancer-related topics (see Useful websites at the end of the chapter).

Dental decay

People with tuberous sclerosis and Down's syndrome and people living with families are more likely to have untreated dental decay (Tiller et al. 2001). When assessing weight loss, aggression at mealtimes and refusal to eat or drink, it is best practice to ensure that teeth and gums are healthy.

Epilepsy

There is a much higher risk of people with learning disabilities having epilepsy, with seizures being harder to control. There are problems with repeated falls and injuries, including additional brain injury and fractures.

Helicobacter pylori

Duff et al. (2001) found high levels of *Helicobacter pylori* in people with learning disabilities living in communal settings; this might be linked to an increased incidence of gastrointestinal cancers.

Incontinence

Both faecal and urinary incontinence have been reported as a problem experienced by older people with learning disabilities (Bland et al. 2003). It is important that there is no diagnostic overshadowing and that people have full access to incontinence services and receive assessment and treatment for their incontinence (DH 2000).

Mobility problems

These are linked to gait problems, physical impairments, joint problems and sensory impairments. In addition, higher levels of foot problems and obesity (Marshall et al. 2003) negatively impact on mobility. People with Down's syndrome are particularly susceptible to atlanto-axial instability – instability of the neck joint that can cause difficulty walking and general weakness. It is good practice to monitor for signs and have yearly checks to ensure there is no deterioration in the neck joint. Poor mobility is significant for older people with learning disabilities as it has implications for changes in living accommodation. Where individuals develop mobility problems, physical causes need to be considered before viewing a 'refusal' to mobilise as challenging behaviour.

Nutrition and weight control

There is a higher risk of obesity or being underweight, with a poor intake of fruit and vegetables, and a poor understanding of healthy eating and suitable activity levels (Messent et al. 1998; Robertson et al. 2000a, 2000b; Marshall et al. 2003). Once identified, proactive health education and support to achieve optimum weight can be beneficial (Marshall et al. 2003), but recommendations need to consider the finances and housing of people and be realistic. Managing nutrition in people with PMLD should include swallowing assessments as they have a higher risk of dysphagia.

Osteoporosis

Aspray et al. (1998) found that people with learning disabilities had lower bone density and a higher risk of fracture, and Jancar and Jancar (1998) found that people with epilepsy were at much higher risk, possibly due to the long-term administration of antiepileptic drugs. Marks et al. (2003) reported that cognitive impairment, dementia and Alzheimer's disease, all of which are more frequent in the learning-disabled population, increase the risk of falls and fractures.

Pain management

Owing to diagnostic overshadowing, inaccurate diagnoses, limited language of pain and poor recognition of pain by carers, pain is often missed or undertreated (Respond 2007). The Disability Distress Assessment Tool has proved useful in identifying pain and monitoring the effectiveness of pain control (Regnard et al. 2007), and is a simple tool that is easy to use.

Polypharmacy

People with learning disabilities have higher incidences of mental illness and challenging behaviour (Cooper et al. 2007), resulting in the long-term use of medication requiring regular review (Deb et al. 2006). As they age and are more likely to be prescribed medication for physical health problems, the monitoring of polypharmacy becomes vital. This is especially important as people with learning disabilities may underreport drug side-effects owing to communication difficulties. Best practice is to have regular reviews and good communication with the prescribing health professionals.

Sensory impairment

Individuals with learning disabilities are between 8.5 and 200 times more likely to have sight impairments and 40% more likely to have hearing loss (Carvill, 2001). Starling et al. (2006) discuss how this is due to the links between eye and brain development and some syndromes including Down's syndrome, fragile X syndrome and cerebral palsy. There is a higher risk of cataracts and multiple sensory losses that affect sight, hearing, taste, smell and touch. Despite this, people are less likely to have a sensory assessment and wear any aids (Starling et al. 2006). Diagnostic overshadowing can be a significant barrier as people attribute behaviours that might indicate sight and hearing loss to the individual's learning disability rather than diminishing sensory ability. With this in mind, it is important that people are encouraged to seek sensory assessments to maximise the vision and hearing they have.

Thyroid disease

There are higher risks especially with people with Down's syndrome, with increasing age being a significant risk factor (Rooney and Walsh 1997).

Partnership working and consent

The first step to good partnership working between client and health professional is gaining informed consent. This requires good communication, accessible information and giving health choices in a manner that supports informed decision-making. The government has published guidance called *Seeking Consent* (DH 2001c), which affirms that people with learning disabilities generally have the capacity to consent and withhold consent, and incapacity must not be assumed. An individual's capacity to consent is not clear cut because a person might be able to consent to less complex health interventions such as cooperating with having a blood pressure check, but lack capacity if a health decision is complex, for example a major operation. It is important that individuals are supported to understand information and make their own choices.

Where health professionals identify that a person does not have the capacity to consent, they are required to provide treatment under 'best interest'. Another adult cannot give consent for a person, but consultation with family, carers and other health professionals might be needed to identify what is in an individual's best interest. It is, however, the health professional's responsibility to make the final best-interest decision. There are resources related to consent and capacity on the DH website, including accessible leaflets about consent to give to people with learning disabilities and their carers. In addition, the Ministry of Justice has a useful *Code of Practice* (2007) to support the Mental Capacity Act 2005 which includes advice on the new mental capacity advocate service, advanced decisions, Lasting Power of Attorney and Court of Protection.

Valuing People (DH 2001a) affirms the importance of partnership working between health professionals and people with learning disabilities. Partners include the person themselves, family members, sometimes friends, and paid care staff working with primary and specialist health professionals. Completing joint annual health assessments between primary care staff and CLDT staff has been piloted by Cassidy et al. (2002), with positive outcomes for individuals. Joint assessment and treatment plans enabled people with learning disabilities and carers to discuss further assessments, treatment options and health complexities, the health professionals being able to contribute different skills to maximise outcomes. This empowers individuals to be active participants in health choices, and Cassidy et al. found that health plans were instigated without the time delays experienced when professionals relied on separate appointments with professional communication *after* appointments. Such partnership working supports good practice as it ensure that plans are acceptable not only to the health professional, but also, most importantly, to the individual (Fender at al. 2007).

Advocacy and empowerment

Rapaport et al. (2005) discuss how devalued groups often turn to advocates for support in presenting their cause. Self-advocates are people able to represent their own needs. If good practice in communication and giving accessible information is followed, the health professional can empower individuals to make informed decisions and develop and implement their own health action plan. However, even with good communication skills, people with learning disabilities might need an advocate to represent their views or support them in some way.

People with learning disabilities access a range of advocates. Rapaport et al. (2005) lists how legal advocates such as lawyers can help when a person's rights are not being upheld, for example an inaccessible public building; collective advocates come together in groups such as MENCAP and People First to fight for the rights of a group of people; peer advocates speak up for individuals with comparable life experiences; and citizen advocates speak up for an individual who needs support. The government is encouraging advocacy projects, but people with learning disabilities can still have problems finding an advocate. Family members often consider they have an advocacy role, as do nurses and social workers. Although these groups can be strong advocates, there can also be conflicts of interest that need acknowledging for the most positive outcome to be reached.

Person-centeredness

For many years, the health needs of people with learning disabilities were provided using a medical model of care. A medical model of care seeks to change or cure the person in isolation from the rest of their life experiences. This model fails to see the person holistically, with their own individual wants and needs and their own social networks and interactions. Person-centred planning is a way of listening to and learning about people so that meaningful choices about their own life are made by the individuals or their carers. This means that people can make their own choices, which their support network can help them achieve. For those with PMLD, it is a way of their networks ensuring good communication and decisions based on a depth of understanding about the individual. By listening carefully, paid carers can help develop a plan that results in an improved quality of life (Hatzidimitriadou and Milne 2005).

Life story work has been shown to have benefits for people with learning disabilities and those who support them. McKeown et al. (2006) discuss how life story books help staff get to know the person, contextualising their behaviours and humanising individuals, and can improve staff attitudes towards individuals and challenge their practice. McKeown et al. acknowledge that developing life stories is a complex task, requiring consent and time, but indicate that staff having the opportunity to do life story work can enrich their practice.

Health assessment

Bland et al. (2003) mentions two effective ways to overcome poor identification and self-reporting of ill-health. The first is to take full opportunity to complete a health assessment whenever health staff have contact with a person. She also suggests that, where opportunities do not arise, it is necessary to arrange health monitoring appointments in a way to encourage attendance. A health assessment might include screening offered to the wider population, but should also include relevant monitoring of health risks specific to people with learning disabilities.

Health action plans

In an effort to reduce inequalities and promote health, the development of health action plans is becoming common practice. These are completed with the individual by practice nurses, learning disability nurses, health trainers or carers. The important thing is that they are accessible and owned by the individual. They can contain medical histories, health education information, health goals, details of medication and a record of meetings with health professionals; they may all be different to reflect the individuality of the person and to meet their communication needs. Having accessible information about the health screening being offered is essential.

End of life care

The Foundation for People with Learning Disabilities published a report in 2002 entitled *Today and Tomorrow: The report of the Growing Older with Learning Disabilities (GOLD) Programme*, which made recommendations for end of life care for older people with learning disabilities. These recommendations were for the prompt diagnosis of terminal illnesses, accessible information supporting an understanding of the treatment options, thoughtful transition from curative interventions to palliative care, person-centred and effective control of symptoms including pain, partnership working including individual, carers and all agencies and services involved in providing support, and support for those who have close relationships with the person who is dying. This final recommendation is essential not only for family members, but also for friends who have learning disabilities and care staff who might have had long-term caring relationships with the individual. Despite these recommendations, Brown et al. (2005) found that people with learning disabilities were continuing to experience diagnostic overshadowing, resulting in slow diagnosis, non-intervention, symptoms being overlooked and a lack of use of hospice or ordinary end of life services. As a consequence, individuals have poor symptom and pain management.

Reflection points

- Reflect upon the end of life and decision-making issues raised in Chapter 3 and the means of communication identified at the beginning of this chapter.
- Then consider how people with mild or moderate learning disabilities could express their end of life needs.
- If they decide to make an advanced decision, who should know of its existence?

Healthcare professionals could recommend the staff or carers to read a publication entitled *Dying Matters* from the Foundation for People with Learning Disabilities (FDLP 2005) to help them understand options and support the person to make informed decisions about their end of life care.

Conclusion

This chapter has explored the factors affecting older people with learning disabilities. Although there is complexity to manage and people with learning disabilities have higher risks of ill-health, being older does not equate to being ill. The aim of health services that support this client group should be apposite assessment, equal and appropriate treatment, and effective partnership working to promote health and reduce the impact of ill-health on quality of life. Well-being is about more than disease management: it is about communication, inclusion, rights, choices and control. Prevention and the early detection of ill-health are key to healthy old age, and people with learning disabilities should be empowered through health education, regular health checks and equality of health treatment to achieve this.

References

Access to Acute (2007) *Access to Acute Care: Supporting People with a Learning Disability on Admission to Hospital.* Available from http://www.nnldn.org.uk/a2a/index.asp.

Aspray, T., Francis, R., Thompson, A., Quilliam, S., Rawlings, D. and Tyrer, S. (1998) Comparison of ultrasound measurements at the heel between adults with mental retardation and control subjects. *Bone* 22(6): 665–8.

Bigby, C. (2005) Growing old: adapting to change and realizing a sense of belonging, continuity and purpose. In G. Grant, P. Goward, M. Richardson and P. Ramcharan (eds.) (2005) *Learning Disability: A Life Cycle Approach to Valuing People.* Maidenhead: Open University Press.

Bland, R., Hutchinson, N., Oakes, P. and Yates, C. (2003) Double jeopardy?: needs and services for older people who have learning disabilities *Journal of Learning Disabilities* 7(4): 323–44.

Brown, H., Flynn, M. and Burns, S. (2005) *Discriminated to Death: Caring for People with Learning Disabilities who are Dying.* Available from http://findarticles.com/p/articles/mi_qa4132/is_200508/ai_n15668158/pg_1?tag=artBody;col1.

Carvill, S. (2001) Sensory impairments, intellectual disability and psychiatry. *Journal of Intellectual Disability Research* 45(6): 467–83.

Cassidy, G., Martin, D., Martin, G. and Roy, A. (2002) Health checks for people with learning disabilities: community learning disability teams working with general practitioners and primary health care teams. *Journal of Intellectual Disabilities* 6(2): 123–36.

Collacott, R., Cooper, S., Branford, D. and McGrother, C. (1998) Behaviour phenotype for Downs syndrome. *British Journal of Psychiatry* 172: 85–9.

Commission for Social Care Inspection (2006) *Joint Investigation into the Provision of Services for People with Learning Disabilities at Cornwall Partnership NHS Trust.* London: CSCI and Healthcare Commission.

Cooper, S. (1997) High prevalence of dementia among people with learning disabilities not attributable to Downs syndrome. *Psychological Medicine* 27(3): 609–16.

Cooper, S., Smiley, E., Morrison, J., Williamson, A. and Allen, L. (2007) Mental ill-health in adults with intellectual disabilities: prevalence and associated factors. *British Journal of Psychiatry* 190: 27–35.

Deb, S., Clarke, D. and Unwin, G. (2006) *Using Medication to Manage Behaviour Problems Among Adults with a Learning Disability. Quick Reference Guide (QRG).* Available from www.LD-Medication.bham.ac.uk.

Department of Health (1998) *Signposts for Success in Commissioning and Providing Health Services for People with Learning Disabilities.* Available from http://www.dh.gov.uk/en/Publicationsandstatistics/Publications/PublicationsPolicyAndGuidance/DH_4008585.

Department of Health (2000) *Good Practice in Continence Services.* Available from http://www.dh.gov.uk/en/Publicationsandstatistics/Publications/PublicationsPolicyAndGuidance/DH_4005851.

Department of Health (2001a) *Valuing People: a New Strategy for Learning Disability for the 21ˢᵗ Century. A White Paper.* Available from http://www.dh.gov.uk/en/Publicationsandstatistics/Publications/PublicationsPolicyAndGuidance/DH_4009153.

Department of Health (2001b) *National Service Framework for Older People.* Available from http://www.dh.gov.uk/en/Publicationsandstatistics/Publications/PublicationsPolicyAndGuidance/DH_4003066.

Department of Health (2001c) *Seeking Consent: Working with People with Learning Disabilities.* Available from http://www.dh.gov.uk/en/Publicationsanstatistics/Publications/PublicationsPolicyAndGuidance/DH_4007861.

Department of Health (2005) *Choosing Health: Making Healthy Choices Easier.* Available from http://www.dh.gov.uk/en/Publicationsandstatistics/Publications/PublicationsPolicyAndGuidance/DH_4094550.

Department of Health (2006) *Our Health, Our Care, Our Say: A New Direction for Community Services.* Available from http://www.dh.gov.uk/en/Publicationsandstatistics/Publications/PublicationsPolicyAndGuidance/DH_4127453.

Department of Health (2007a) *Human Rights in Healthcare – a Framework for Local Action.* Available from http://www.dh.gov.uk/en/Publicationsandstatistics/Publications/PublicationsPolicyAndGuidance/DH_073473.

Department of Health (2007b) *Primary Care Service Framework: Management of Health for People with Learning Disabilities in Primary Care.* Available from http://www.primarycarecontracting.nhs.uk/uploads/primary_care_service_frameworks/primary_care_service_framework__ld_v3_final.pdf.

Disability Rights Commission (2006) *Equal Treatment: Closing the Gap.* Available from http://www.library.nhs.uk/mentalhealth/ViewResource.aspx?resID=187303.

Djuretic, T., Laing-Morton, T., Guy, M. and Gill, M. (1999) Concerted effort is needed to ensure these women use preventative services. *British Medical Journal* 316(7182): 537.

Doody, G.A., Gotz, M., Johnstone, E.C., Frith, C.D. and Owens, D.G. (1998) Theory of mind and psychoses. *Psychological Medicine* 28(2): 397–405.

Duff, M., Hoghton, M., Scheepers, M., Cooper, M. and Baddeley, P. (2001) *Helicobacter pylori*: has the killer escaped from the institution? A possible cause of increased stomach cancer in a population with learning disabilities. *Journal of Intellectual Disability Research* 45(3): 219–25.

Emerson, E., Hatton, C., Felce, D. and Murphy, G. (2001) *Learning Disability: The Fundamental Facts.* London: Mental Health Foundation.

Fender, A., Marsden, L. and Starr, J. (2007) Assessing the health of older adults with intellectual disabilities. *Journal of Intellectual Disabilities* 11(3): 223–39.

Forbat, L. (2006) An analysis of key principles in valuing people: implications for supporting people with dementia. *Journal of Intellectual Disabilities* 10(3): 249–60.

Forbat, L. and Wilkinson, H. (2008) Where should people with dementia live? Using views of service users to inform models of care. *British Journal of Learning Disabilities* 36(1): 6–12.

Foundation for People with Learning Disabilities (2001) *Misplaced and Forgotten: People with Learning Disabilities in Residential Services for Older People.* London: Mental Health Foundation.

Foundation for People with Learning Disabilities (2002) *Today and Tomorrow: the Report of the Growing Older with Learning Disabilities Programme (GOLD).* Available from http://www.learningdisabilities.org.uk/our-work/personcentred-support/gold/.

Foundation for People with Learning Disabilities (2005) *Dying Matters.* Available at http://www.learningdisabilities.org.uk.

Gloucestershire Partnership NHS Trust (2005) *Traffic Light Assessment: Red Amber Green, Hospital Assessment for People with Learning Disabilities.* Gloucester: Gloucestershire Partnership NHS Trust.

Hassiotis, A., Barron, P. and O'Hara, J. (2000) Mental health services for people with learning disabilities: a complete overhaul is needed with strong links to mainstream services. *British Medical Journal* 321(7261): 583–4.

Hatzidimitriadou, E. and Milne, A. (2005) Planning ahead, meeting the needs of older people with intellectual disabilities in the UK. *Dementia* 4(3): 341–55.

Hemmings, C. and Greig, A. (2007) Mental health or learning disabilities? The use of a specialist inpatient unit for a man with learning disabilities, schizophrenia and vascular dementia. *Advances in Mental Health and Learning Disabilities* 1(2): 32–5.

Hermon, C., Alberman, E., Beral, V. and Swerdlow, A. (2001) Mortality and cancer incidence in persons with Downs syndrome their parents and siblings. *Annals of Human Genetics* 65(2): 167–76.

Holland, A., Hon, J., Huppert, F., Stevens, S. and Watson, P. (1998) Population based study of the prevalence and presentation of dementia in adults with Downs syndrome. *British Journal of Psychiatry* 172: 493–8.

Hollins, S., Attard, M.T., Von Fraunhofer, N., McGuigan, S. and Sedgwick, P. (1998) Mortality in people with learning disability: risks, causes and death certification findings in London. *Developmental Medicine and Child Neurology* 40(1): 50–6.

Jancar, J. (1998) The problems of ageing. In C. Hallas, W. Fraser, D. Sines and M. Kerr (eds.) *Hallas' The Care of People With Intellectual Disabilities*, 9th edn. Oxford: Butterworth Heinemann.

Jancar, J. and Jancar, M. (1998) Age related fractures in people with intellectual disability and epilepsy. *Journal of Intellectual Disability Research* 42(5): 429–33.

Jones, J. (2001) *The Communication Gap.* Available from http://www.somerset.gov.uk/somerset/socialservices/pi/stc/.

Kerr, A.M., McCulloch, D., Oliver, K. et al. (2003) Medical needs of people with intellectual disability require regular reassessment, and the provision of client- and carer-held reports. *Journal of Intellectual Disability Research* 47(2): 134–45.

Kirk, L., Hick, R. and Laraway, A. (2006) Assessing dementia in people with learning disabilities: the relationship between two screening measures. *Journal of Intellectual Disabilities* 10(4): 357–64.

McKeown, J., Clarke, A. and Repper, J. (2006) Life story work in health and social care: a systematic literature review. *Journal of Advanced Nursing* 55(2): 237–47.

Marks, R., Allegrante, J.P., Ronald MacKenzie, C. and Lane, J.M. (2003) Hip fractures among the elderly; causes, consequences and control. *Ageing Research Reviews* 2(1): 57–93.

Marshall, D., McConkey, R. and Moore, G. (2003) Obesity in people with intellectual disabilities: the impact of nurse-led health screening and health promotion activities. *Journal of Advanced Nursing* 41(2): 147–53.

MENCAP (2003a) *Treat Me Right – Better Healthcare for People with a Learning Disability.* Available from http://www.library.nhs.uk/learningdisabilities/ViewResource.aspx?resID=51823.

MENCAP (2003b) *Breaking Point.* Available from http://www.mencap.org.uk/document.asp?id=297.

MENCAP (2007a) *Death by Indifference.* Available from http://www.mencap.org.uk/document.asp?id=284.

MENCAP (2007b) *PMLD Definition.* Available from http://www.mencap.org.uk/document.asp?id=2345.

Messent, P., Cooke, C. and Long, J. (1998) Physical activity, exercise and health of adults with mild and moderate learning disabilities. *British Journal of Learning Disabilities* 26(1): 17–22.

Ministry of Justice (2007) *Mental Capacity Act (2005): Code of Practice.* Available from http://www.justice.gov.uk/docs/mca-cp-plain1.pdf.

People First. Available at http://www.peoplefirstltd.com.

Plimley, L. (2007) A review of quality of life issues and people with autism spectrum disorders. *British Journal of Learning Disabilities* 35(4): 205–13.

Rapaport, J., Manthorpe, J., Moriarty, J., Hussein, S. and Collins, J. (2005) Advocacy and people with learning disabilities in the UK: how can local funders find value for money? *Journal of Intellectual Disabilities* 9(4): 299–320.

Read, S. and Elliott, D. (2007) Exploring the continuum of support for bereaved people with intellectual disabilities: a strategic approach. *Journal of Intellectual Disabilities* 11(2): 167–82.

Regnard, C., Reynolds, J., Watson, B., Matthews, D., Gibson, L. and Clarke, C. (2007) Understanding distress in people with severe communication difficulties: developing and assessing the Disability Distress Assessment Tool (DisDAT). *Journal of Intellectual Disability Research* 51(4): 277–92.

Respond (2007) *People with Learning Disability – an Ageing Population.* Available from www.respond.org.uk/support/resources/articles/people_with_learning_disabilities-_an_ageing_population.html.

Robertson, J., Emerson, E., Gregory, N. et al. (2000a). Lifestyle related risk factors for poor health in residential settings for people with intellectual disabilities. *Research in Developmental Disabilities* 21(6): 469–86.

Robertson, J., Emerson, E., Gregory, N., Hatto, C., Kessissoglou, S. and Hallam, A. (2000b) Receipt of psychotropic medication by people with intellectual disability in residential settings. *Journal of Intellectual Disability Research* 44(Pt 6): 666–76.

Rooney, S. and Walsh, E. (1997) Prevalence of abnormal thyroid function tests in a Down's syndrome population. *Irish Journal of Medical Science* 166(2): 80–2.

Rose, I. (2006) *All About Me*. Luton: Luton and Dunstable Hospital.

Scarborough, K. (2008) *Health Trainers with Learning Disabilities*. Presentation at Learning, Teaching and Assessing Committee, University of the West of England.

Scope (2007) *An Introduction to Ageing and Cerebral Palsy*. Milton Keynes: Scope.

Smiley, E. (2005) Epidemiology of mental health problems in adults with learning disability: an update. *Advances in Psychiatric Treatment* 11: 214–22,.

Starling, S., Willis, A., Dracup, M., Burton, M. and Pratt, C. (2006) Right to Sight Accessing eye care for adults who are learning disabled. *Journal of Intellectual Disabilities* 10(4): 337–55.

Strydom, A. and Hassiotis, A. (2003) Diagnostic instruments for dementia in older people with intellectual disability in clinical practice. *Ageing and Mental Health* 7(6): 431–7.

Sullivan, S., Hussain, R., Threlfall, T. and Bittles, A. (2005) The incidence of cancer in people with intellectual disabilities. *Cancer Causes and Control* 15(10): 1021–5.

Thompson, D. (2002) Growing older with learning disabilities. *Journal of Learning Disabilities* 6(2): 115–22.

Tiller, S., Wilson, K. and Gallagher, J. (2001) Oral health status and dental service use of adults with learning disabilities living in residential institutions and in the community. *Community Dental Health* 18(3): 167–71.

Whittell, B. and Ramcharan, P. (2000) The trouble with kids: an account of problems experienced with local children by people with learning disabilities. *British Journal of Learning Disabilities* 28(1): 21–4.

World Health Organization (1996) *ICD-10 Guide for Mental Retardation*. Available from http://www.who.int/mental_health/media/en/69.pdf.

Wilkinson, H., Kerr, D., Cunningham, C. and Rae, C. (2004) *Support for People with Learning Difficulties in Residential Settings who Develop Dementia*. York: Joseph Rowntree Foundation.

Xenitidis, K., Gratsa, A., Bouras, N. et al. (2003) Psychiatric inpatient care for adults with intellectual disabilities: generic or specialist units? *Journal of Intellectual Disability Research* 48(1): 11–18.

Useful websites

CHANGE: http://www.intellectualdisability.info/home.htm
National Network for Learning Disability Nurses: http://www.nnldn.org.uk

Chapter 6

Working with older people with dementia in the community

Mary Marshall

Introduction

This chapter aims to show how challenging and rewarding it is to work with people with dementia and their carers who live in the community. It can be no more than an introduction to key issues. The text covers the policy context, dementia from a medical and social point of view, ethical and philosophical concerns, communication, working with other professionals and organisations, and challenges and rewards.

What is dementia?

There is no simple answer to the question 'what is dementia?' Dementia is very different for each individual. If we are to be truly person centred, this is where we have to start. We start with the person who is on the journey and those who travel alongside, who may be relatives or friends and can, for periods of this journey, be paid staff. Very occasionally, a professional can be with the person and the carers for the whole journey, and this can be very helpful. This chapter will use the word 'carers' for family and friends; words like 'paid staff', 'professionals', etc. will be used for those who are involved through their work. The experience of dementia is profoundly affected by the degree to which cognitive skills are important to the person, the kind of person they are, the kind of relationships they have, their physical health and so on.

We also have to be aware of our own attitudes and the way they can stand in the way of truly understanding what individuals are experiencing.

For many of us, the thought of losing memory and cognitive competence is truly terrifying, and we can bring this fear and anxiety to the situation. We can fail to see the remaining competencies, the potential and the rewards (Bryden 2005). Steven Post puts it very clearly:

> In our hyper-cognitive culture and society . . . nothing is as fearful as Alzheimer's Disease (AD) because it violates the spirit of self-control, independence, economic productivity, and cognitive enhancement that defines our dominant image of human fulfilment. . . . the hyper-cognitive societies . . . can neglect the emotional, relational, aesthetic and spiritual aspects of well-being. (2000: 245)

He is surely correct in his assertion that we can neglect the emotional, relational, aesthetic and spiritual aspects of well-being, which means we neglect the abilities that people with dementia retain much longer than their cognitive function.

Reflection points

- Consider a patient with dementia and the extent to which his or her capacity for creativity was assessed.

Before we look at the medical and social understandings of dementia, we need to consider the policy context and the roles in which nurses in the community may encounter people with dementia and their carers.

Policy context

In England, and to some extent in the other devolved governments of the UK, there has recently been a surge of reports about dementia, culminating in dementia becoming a National Health Service priority, and the formulation of a dementia strategy consultation in 2008. The Alzheimer's Society (2007) produced a powerful report of data about prevalence, costs and projections for the future. In 2006, the National Institute for Health and Clinical Excellence (NICE) and the Social Care Institute for Excellence (SCIE) produced clinical guidelines, and in 2007 the National Audit Office (NAO) published the report *Improving Services and Support for Older People with Dementia* recommending early diagnosis. The momentum was to some extent generated by previous reports such as the Audit Commission's influential reports *Forget me Not* (2002, 2000), *The National Service Framework for Older People* (Department of Health [DH] 2001) and, to some extent for mental illness, the Care Services

Improvement Partnership (CSIP) service development guide *Everybody's Business* (2005). Not all of these are specifically about dementia, but they have been major steps towards a *National Dementia Strategy* for England (DH 2008).

The dementia strategy has three main themes: improving awareness and diminishing stigma; early diagnosis so that interventions can start early; and a high quality of care and support. There is a determination to put the person with dementia and their carers in control, which is a recurring principle in this chapter.

Roles for nurses in the community

A study conducted by Bryans et al. (2003) identified that practitioners working in primary care were not confident in diagnosing dementia or working with people and their families who had received such a diagnosis. Nolan et al. (2002) noted that some healthcare workers found working with people with dementia in primary care a less than satisfying and positive experience, as they felt unprepared and were challenged by their lack of knowledge of dementia and its effects on the older person and their family. People working in the community setting have an important role when working with people with dementia as they provide a link between primary and secondary care and, ideally, continuity of care from the point of diagnosis to end of life care (Manthorpe and Illiffe 2007).

Nurses come into contact with people with dementia living in the community as district nurses, practice nurses, health visitors, community psychiatric nurses and nursing assistants. They may also be running community resources such as day centres and day hospitals, clubs or groups. Nurses are also employed by local authorities as care managers. Many residential and nursing homes are run by nurses, especially those that specialise in dementia care. They may be attached to a memory clinic or a research project.

In these various professional roles, there may be several reasons why nurses are in touch with the person with dementia:

- *doing an assessment*: usually either prior to referral for diagnosis, as part of a single shared assessment or as a specialist assessment
- *providing information*: people with dementia and their carers always say, when asked, that they do not have enough information. This is not as straightforward as it sounds. Information is required of the right sort, in the right language, in the right amounts and at the right time
- *counselling and support*: again, this can concern issues of diagnosis, relationships or sexual difficulties, or it might simply be listening and encouraging
- *advising on behaviour problems*: especially in care homes

- *coordinating, linking and advocating*: in relation to services
- *providing a service*: to small or large groups of people with dementia.

The medical view of dementia

It is easy to stereotype the medical view of dementia as being primarily concerned with the brain, but for ease of explanation we will stay with this view for the moment. Medical diagnoses are standardised in various ways. Here we will use the *International Classification of Diseases 10th Revision* classification (World Health Organization 1990):

> Dementia is a syndrome due to disease of the brain, usually of a chronic or progressive nature, in which there is a disturbance of multiple higher cortical functions, including memory, thinking, orientation, comprehension, calculation, learning capacity, language and judgement. Impairments of cognitive function are commonly accompanied and occasionally preceded by deterioration in emotional control, social behaviour, or motivation.

The term 'dementia' is used for a cluster of chronic or progressive diseases of the brain. The Alzheimer's Society website gives very good basic information (see Useful websites at the end of the chapter), and the fact sheets numbered below can be found on there. The website says, 'There are several diseases and conditions that cause dementia.' These include:

- *Alzheimer's disease*: – 'The most common cause of dementia. During the course of the disease the chemistry and structure of the brain changes, leading to the death of brain cells' (Factsheet 401, *What is Alzheimer's Disease?*). It is really not possible to make a firm diagnosis until a post mortem, when it is clear that there are numerous serial plaques, neurofibrillary tangles and beta-amyloid protein deposits (Nagy and Hubbard 2008).
- *Vascular disease*: 'The brain relies on a network of vessels to bring it oxygen-bearing blood. If the oxygen supply to the brain fails, brain cells are likely to die and this can cause the symptoms of vascular dementia. These symptoms can occur either suddenly, following a stroke, or over time through a series of small strokes' (Factsheet 402, *What is Vascular Dementia?*).
- *Dementia with Lewy bodies*: 'This form of dementia gets its name from tiny spherical structures that develop inside nerve cells. Their presence in the brain leads to the degeneration of brain tissue. Memory, concentration and language skills are affected. This form of dementia shares some characteristics with Parkinson's disease' (Factsheet 403, *What is Dementia with Lewy Bodies (DLB)?*).

- *Fronto-temporal dementia (including Pick's disease)*: 'In fronto-temporal dementia, damage is usually focused in the front part of the brain. At first, personality and behaviour are more affected than memory' (Factsheet 404, *What is Fronto-temporal Dementia (Including Pick's Disease)?*).

As can be seen from the fact sheets, each type of dementia has a different progression, although this is by no means clear cut. Indeed, nothing is clear cut in the dementia world: there is even an ongoing controversy among scientists about whether these are 'diseases' or whether they are a consequence of ageing and some of us age faster than others (Anderson 2008). The other complication is that many people have a combination of Alzheimer's disease and vascular dementia. It is increasingly clear that there is a degree of overlap in all dementias (Holmes 2008). In very general terms, Alzheimer's disease progresses slowly, whereas vascular dementia progresses in steps. The majority, about 50%, of people who have dementia will have Alzheimer's disease.

Many people with dementia and their carers will want to talk about the causes of dementia: 'Why me?,' they may say. There is no clear answer. The normal things that cause arteriosclerotic damage, such as diet, smoking and lack of exercise, will impact on dementia. The scientists looking at prevention seem to be saying that the lead-time is really long and that the risk factors need to be addressed as long as 20–30 years earlier. Age itself is obviously a risk factor. The proportion of older people with dementia increases with age. Educational level is another risk factor, although this may be to do with lifestyle factors for people with poor educational achievement (Frataglioni et al. 2008).

Another dementia, which is not in the list above because it can be to some degree treated, is alcohol-related brain damage (ARBD) On the Alzheimer's Society web page, this is called Korsakoff's disease. This is caused by prolonged abuse of alcohol and the resulting lack of thiamine (vitamin B1). A good diet can help people with ARBD regain some competence but often have a chronically impaired memory. The number of people with ARBD is increasing, and they can present particular problems because of their lifestyle and history, and because many of them are relatively young. Alcohol is also a complicating factor for many people with other dementias (O'Connell and Lawler 2008).

Reflection points

- **People with ARBD are rarely considered to have dementia and to be in need of the same quality of care. Why might this be?**

The Alzheimer's Society website lists the following things people can do to prevent dementia:

- Don't smoke
- Reduce your intake of saturated fat
- Take regular exercise
- Drink alcohol in moderation
- Eat a healthy diet and maintain a normal body weight
- Eat plenty of fruit and vegetables, particularly those that contain vitamin C or vitamin A
- Eat oily fish once a week
- Have a GP check your blood pressure and cholesterol levels
- Avoid head injuries (wear a helmet for cycling or motorcycling, and don't box)
- Have an active social life, outside interests and hobbies

People with dementia and their carers will sometimes want to talk about how long they have to live, and again the answer is not clear. Most people with dementia will die of something else but the dementia will shorten their life. Some people, who are in good health when they get dementia, can live for well over 10 years.

People with dementia and their carers may also want to talk about the extent to which it is inherited. For some younger people (those aged under 60), there seems to be a clear genetic factor in that it seems to run in some families. People with Down's syndrome are particularly at risk of Alzheimer's disease in their middle age. The Down's Syndrome Association web page says that the incidence is about the same as for the general population but that it occurs 20–30 years earlier. (See Chapter 5 for a further discussion.) The number of younger people with dementia is not large (about 15,000 in England according to the 2007 NAO report), but it can be very traumatic since they may have jobs and young families and be otherwise in good health. Genetic factors are less clear for older people, so on the whole health carers can reassure the families of older people that it is by no means certain they will get it.

As these are diseases of the brain, there are symptoms affecting some people that result from brain damage and that may need to be explained:

- *Visual agnosia*: the inability to recognise familiar objects
- *Prosopagnosia*: the inability to recognise faces
- *Object agnosia*: the inability to name objects
- *Colour agnosia*: the inability to discriminate between colours and therefore to name them
- *Apraxia of speech*: the person has difficulty saying what he or she wants to say correctly and consistently
- *Aphasia*: a complex disorder of language and communication that is subdivided into three sections:

1. *Anomia* – the inability to access spoken names for objects, most often associated with the older person or those with brain damage to the left hemisphere. People with anomia often use circumlocutions (speaking in a roundabout way) in order to express a certain word whose name they cannot remember. Sometimes the person can recall the name when given clues. Individuals are often frustrated when they know that they know the name but cannot produce it.

2. *Paraphrasia* – saying a word that sounds like another word, or saying a word that is related but a different idea, for instance 'lips' for 'hips' or 'latch' instead of 'match'. Individuals with cortical types of dementia, like Alzheimer's disease, do this a lot. Sometimes it might sound confusing, and one will need to be very patient to try to understand what the person is trying to explain.

3. *Agrammatism* – people with dementia have difficulty ordering words and putting them together in a coherent sentence. Words or endings of words may be omitted from a sentence, or the connections between the words may not be included, so the sentence becomes a series of apparently unrelated words, for example girl, biscuit and water. This makes little sense without the connecting words for this sentence, i.e. the girl slipped on the water and dropped her biscuit.

- *Perseveration*: repeatedly carrying out the same activity, making the same gesture or asking the same question.

The medical model can be seen as a rather gloomy one in that there is very little that can be done about brain damage. There are drugs which, for a minority, can slow down the development of Alzheimer's disease for a time. These are the cholinesterase inhibitors donepezil (Aricept), galantamine (Reminyl) and rivastigmine (Exelon). There has been a lot of controversy about these drugs because the NICE Technology Appraisal (2007) said they should only be used for the middle stages, a decision opposed by many of the organisations concerned with people with dementia. It may need to be explained to those with dementia and their carers that these drugs only help a minority of people, so they should not be disappointed if they are not prescribed for them or they do not work for particular individuals.

Professionals may also find themselves having to explain that the successful treatments people read about constantly in the papers take many years to test fully, so they themselves are unlikely to benefit. There is a great deal of research being undertaken at present, and it is a good idea to monitor the Alzheimer's Society website to ensure that advice imparted is sound. Some people will want to talk to nurses about alternative therapies such as ginkgo biloba, for which the evidence is inconclusive. They should be advised to talk to their GP if they are considering alternative medicines. It may be useful to remember that research by Brooker and Woolley (2006) indicated that activity programmes have success rates equivalent to those of medication without any side-effects, so these can be recommended.

There are also drugs that can be given to control some of the accompanying behaviours, but these are not usually recommended and we will look at this issue later in the section on behaviour.

Conditions often confused with dementia: delirium and depression

Many older people are depressed (Manthorpe and Illiffe 2005), and severe depression can easily be mistaken for dementia (Cunningham et al. 2007). A careful history will usually reveal the differences. As highlighted in Chapter 4, it is important to note that people with dementia can have a depression, which often goes unrecognised; and this is not just in the early stages. Nurses have an important role in recognising depression. Olin et al. (2002) have produced guidelines for the diagnosis of depression in people with dementia and stress symptoms such as reduced positive affect, social isolation and withdrawal. The GP should be consulted and medication considered. More activities and improved social interaction may also help. The Alzheimer's Society web page is helpful on both depression and delirium.

Delirium is a matter of serious concern in terms of the number of times it is mistaken for dementia and the wrong treatment given (Manning 2003). Delirium results from an acute infection, high levels of stress or pain for example, and its symptoms are of sudden onset. The community nurse may need to share his or her knowledge of the person in the community to ensure others recognise that this is not the person's usual behaviour. The treatment should be of the underlying condition, such as the infection. The most worrying kind of delirium occurs in the person who becomes very quietly confused and may actually be very ill, but since they are causing no problem, they are not treated quickly enough. Delirium should be assumed for any sudden change of competence, mood or behaviour, and nurses will have a particularly important role in working out what the cause may be and how best to treat it (Hogg 2008).

Reflection points

- Why do you think that delirium is so often misdiagnosed?
- Is there anything that could be done to improve the accuracy of diagnosis and treatment?

The social view of dementia

The social view of dementia takes the brain damage as a fact but suggests that much of the experience and expression of dementia relate to the *interaction* between individuals with impairments and their social and built environment. This is most easily explained using a diagram (Figure 6.1).

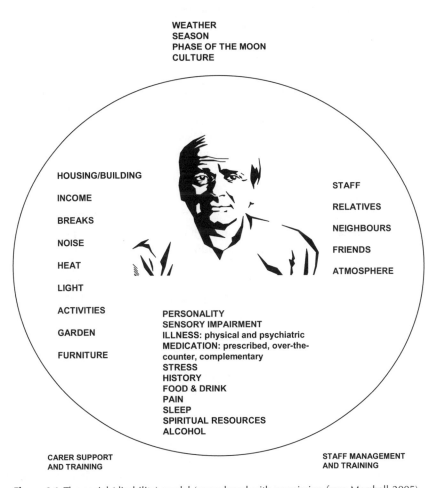

The Social (Disability) Model

WEATHER
SEASON
PHASE OF THE MOON
CULTURE

HOUSING/BUILDING

INCOME

BREAKS

NOISE

HEAT

LIGHT

ACTIVITIES

GARDEN

FURNITURE

STAFF

RELATIVES

NEIGHBOURS

FRIENDS

ATMOSPHERE

PERSONALITY
SENSORY IMPAIRMENT
ILLNESS: physical and psychiatric
MEDICATION: prescribed, over-the-counter, complementary
STRESS
HISTORY
FOOD & DRINK
PAIN
SLEEP
SPIRITUAL RESOURCES
ALCOHOL

CARER SUPPORT
AND TRAINING

STAFF MANAGEMENT
AND TRAINING

Figure 6.1 The social (disability) model (reproduced with permission from Marshall 2005).

This gentleman has brain damage. His experience of dementia will be affected by all the things that are below him in the figure – his past life, his health and so on, and all the items surrounding him. Things in the larger world such as weather and culture will also impact on his experience. This is a more positive view than the medical view because there is a great deal that can be done to improve the social and the built environment to optimise the experience for individuals and their carers.

The citizenship view

This is a more contemporary way of thinking which suggests that the experts in dementia are the people who have it. They need to be taken seriously as people who have both rights and responsibilities. They have a right to a diagnosis, a right to be heard and a right to participate as far as they are able (Innes et al. 2004). Citizenship is about reciprocity, and people with dementia should be expected (and enabled) to make a contribution: to give gifts, to help others, to create if they have the talent and so on.

Clearly, this view is easier to understand for people who are not too disabled by the disease, but as professionals we can ensure that we hold this view even for more disabled people. People with dementia retain a wish to communicate, and this will be covered later in the chapter.

Stages of dementia

You may have noticed that this chapter has not described the 'stages of dementia', which have been codified in different ways (see Alzheimer's Society and British Medical Journal websites at the end of the chapter). This is because anticipating stages can blind us to the uniqueness of every person's journey. Yes, these are progressive diseases, and people become more disabled as they journey, but their personal pathway is unique because the experience of dementia is affected by so many things.

Philosophical and ethical concerns

Language

We need to be very careful about the language we use. 'People with dementia' prefer this term to 'demented people' or 'dementia sufferers' in that they want us to see the person before we see the dementia. Alzheimer Europe prefers 'people living with dementia'. Some people really dislike the word 'dementia', and in the USA the word Alzheimer's disease is used to cover most of the dementias. In the UK, we have 'Alzheimer's societies', which can lead people with other dementias to think they are not eligible for help.

Describing the behaviour of people with dementia without being pejorative is important although not easy. 'Challenging behaviour' is a term much used because it does not say for whom it is challenging. Some people prefer 'behaviour which challenges'. Others refuse to use either term because they would not use language like that with other adults. Describing the actual behaviour also presents problems. It has been acceptable for too long to use words that, in effect, blame people with dementia (Marshall and Allan 2006). Terms such as 'wandering', 'resistant' and 'aggressive' are very negative and fail to address the issue that the problem may actually be with the staff or relative and not with the person with dementia – although it is, of course, most likely to be a combination of these. It is better to be detailed as we would be with other adults and to use terms like 'walking' and 'angry', which force us to be more specific and careful. Another problematic term is 'respite', which can be felt to be very offensive to people with dementia. Why should my relative need respite from me? A better term is 'breaks', but the word respite persists in common usage.

Seeing the person

The term 'person-centred care' so lucidly explained in relation to people with dementia by Kitwood (1997) is by no means an easy aspiration. Brooker (2008) comments that the challenge for this century is whether it is possible to make person-centred care a reality in everyday practice. To focus on the individual when there are so many competing demands is very hard. It is easier to do this in the community than in institutions (Alzheimer's Society 2001) because there are many reminders of the person's identity and we are seeing them in context, but it is still difficult. Ideally, it means that we know the person with dementia well. We know their history, their preferences, their beliefs and their families, and they are in control as far as possible. We do nothing to diminish them as people and citizens.

Seeing the relationships

Increasingly, in the professional literature, we are seeing a focus on relationships (Nolan 2004; Nolan et al. 2008). Few of us can live without them, and it is the role of professionals to understand and support them. And this is not just in the practical sense. We derive a lot of our view of ourselves from the quality of our relationships. We have, in community care, tended to see the needs of people with disabilities and those of their carers as separate. Indeed, this is enshrined in legislation. In fact, however, we need to focus more often on the relationship itself (Robinson et al. 2005). Adams (2008: 107) refers to this as 'dyadic approaches towards dementia care nursing'. Interestingly, he goes on to mention 'triadic approaches' (p. 120), in which, with the professional, a group of three is formed. He suggests that triangular relationships are inherently difficult, which may explain why it can be very hard to see both individuals with dementia and their carers as partners in care at the same time. Nolan et al. (2008) provide a useful senses framework for relationship-centred care in care homes: a sense of security, a sense of belonging and so on.

Discrimination and stigma

People with dementia face a double discrimination – first because they are older, and second, because they have a disease of the brain and experience all the stigma that people with mental health problems experience. In the *National Dementia Strategy* Consultation (DH 2008), the Secretary of State specifically mentions the need to remove stigma. People with dementia often say that they can cope with the dementia but not with the stigma. They are living with a disease that terrifies many professionals and policy-makers, and they are one of a great many (700,000 in the UK, 570,000 in England). The net result is that most policy-makers put dementia into the '*too difficult*' basket, and it is only very recently that it has been made any sort of policy priority. This means that our role as professionals can be very difficult. We can find ourselves fighting constant battles for some degree of fairness in the distribution of services or in the quality of services. This is not a field of work for the faint-hearted.

A rehabilitation approach

This is another way of describing a more positive attitude to dementia care and one that is well understood in health services. It is increasingly common to hear reference to 'rehabilitation', both in the general sense and specifically in relation to people with dementia who have had acute psychiatric or physical interventions (Marshall 2005). It suggests that we need to help people achieve their optimum function and quality of life, and that there is much we can do. Huusko et al. (2000) undertook a randomised control trial which showed that people with dementia who had had an acute hospital intervention responded significantly to individually tailored rehabilitation. This is an important finding because they are often at the end, rather than the beginning, of the queue. There is currently much research into cognitive rehabilitation, especially for people in the earlier stages of dementia (Clare 2005).

Conflicts of interest

There can be real conflicts of interest between the needs of people with dementia and the needs of their families and friends. There can also be conflicts of interest between the needs of people with dementia and those of responsible professionals such as GPs or community mental health nurses. Nobody wants people with dementia to come to harm or be blamed if things go wrong. This relates to risk, which is increasingly an issue of concern in our risk-averse, blame culture (Adams 2001). There is a lot of comforting talk from managers about risk assessment, but this is an art and not a science (Manthorpe 2003). This is not to say that nurses in the community should not have clearly assessed the risks to the person and done what they can to achieve a balance between quality of life and minimising risk (Thom and Blair 1998; Dewing and Blackburn 1999; Gilmour 2004; Titterton 2004). Nurses should bear in mind that they have a professional duty to promote autonomy wherever possible (Nursing and Midwifery Council 2008). Risks such as cognitive deterioration from boredom, and depression from loss of control of one's life, are rarely considered because the impact is invisible. Risk assessments need to be in writing and need to be shared.

> **Reflection points**
>
> - When did you last assess a person with dementia as being at risk of deterioration because he or she was bored?
> - What were you able to do about this risk?

Moments of lucidity

Very disabled people with dementia can have moments of lucidity, which can be very disturbing for carers and care staff who are left wondering whether the person really has a dementia. They may feel very guilty about the way they have related to the person. These moments of lucidity are now the subject of research (Norman et al. 2006). Reassurance that they happen to other people can be very helpful.

Spirituality

Spirituality is hard to define. For some it means religion, for others it means person-centred care, and it can mean those aspects of life that are beyond the day to day. One of the problems is that the term will mean different things to different people. For the religious, the opportunity for familiar worship can be absolutely essential, and we need to bear in mind the number of different religions and different traditions within each religion. There are important theological considerations relating to dementia, such as the nature of the soul when memory has gone, and there are now some useful books on the subject (Goldsmith 2004). Some people will understand person-centred care better if it is couched in the language of spirituality, which for them will be about the essential uniqueness of each individual. For others, spirituality is about nature or music or art. Feeling the rain on your face or being near a tree is life enhancing for some people. Others may have a favourite style of music that nurtures them more than anything else. 'Spirituality' is a term to be used carefully but not avoided. In one way or other it is important to everybody.

Communication

Verbal communication: one-to-one

People with dementia are usually really grateful if you say who you are when you meet, even if you have met before. We all get embarrassed at being unable to remember names, but for people with dementia this is a very common experience. We need to say who we are and why we are there. A clear name badge can be helpful.

People with dementia tend to be older, which means that many will have impaired hearing and eyesight that make listening to what you are saying difficult. They may be unable to understand why they cannot make sense of what you are saying. They may also be very anxious. Choosing a quiet, familiar place for the conversation, ensuring there is plenty of light, sitting on a level with or slightly below the person and speaking clearly will help. It may be necessary to check that hearing aids are working or that spectacles have been found. It is also important to bear in mind that most people with dementia have impaired memory and impaired reasoning, so asking direct questions can be very harassing for them. It is better to give some prompts and suggestions in a gentle way, and to keep the questions simple and short. Many people with dementia will not even be able to manage this and will prefer a conversation instead. If this is the case, it is important to remember that people with dementia will often tell you what they are feeling through stories and metaphors. Thus, when they say they want to go home to collect the children from school, what they may be saying is that they want to be busy and to be significant to others. Many of the communication strategies and tips suggested in Chapter 5 will work equally well with a person with dementia.

It can sometimes help to ask indirect questions to get an opinion or a preference (Allan 2001). Thus, one might say, 'What would you say to someone who was thinking of having help with bathing?' Or one might involve someone in a photograph: 'What would your mother think of me bandaging your leg ulcers?' In more organised consultations with groups of people with dementia (McAndrew and Taylor 2006), it can be very helpful to have a large sheet of paper in front of the group and to draw reminders of what has been talked about. This technique is well used with people with learning disabilities and has also been found to work well with people with dementia.

It is worth remembering that people whose first language is not English may forget their English and be able to communicate only in their native tongue. Sometimes speech impairment is assumed when the problem is actually the need for an interpreter.

Reflection points

- How might you advise an interpreter to assist you in your communication with a person with dementia whose language you cannot speak?

Verbal communication: in groups

There is an increasing literature about group work with people with dementia, that is, small groups with the same membership throughout. These groups seem to allow their members to feel in control and confident about sharing their feelings (Cheston et al. 2003; Bender 2004). Many nurses in day hospitals run similar groups. There are important skills in making sure that the groups are started and finished carefully and that the leaders (and there are usually two) have time for a debriefing. Support groups with an information purpose are rarely used for people with dementia but are common for groups of carers.

Non-verbal communication

Crisp (2003) rightly reminds us that everything that is said or done by nurses communicates something about their attitudes to those in their care. People with dementia can be very finely tuned to non-verbal communication (Scenarios 6.1 and 6.2). It is really important to reflect on what your body language is saying. Is it saying, 'I am too busy to sit down and talk to you', or 'I find you repellent so I am not sitting close to you'?

Scenario 6.1: Non-verbal communication

Mr McIntosh was almost unable to speak, but when I put my cheek against his and held his hand, I could hear that, in response to my question, he was saying was that he liked the nursing home and the food was good.

Scenario 6.2: Body language

Joan was asked to bath Mrs Lloyd, who was in bed. She approached with a basin of hot water and a flannel, and pulled back the bedclothes. She was horrified when Mrs Lloyd screamed and writhed away. After training, Joan learned that she should put the water on the floor and should sit down herself, making eye contact with Mrs Lloyd. She learned to talk gently, working her way round to mentioning a wash. She started offering to wash Mrs Lloyd's face, which was a bit sticky. Mrs Lloyd was relaxed and enjoyed that. Talking gently all the time, and allowing Mrs Lloyd to be in charge as much as possible, made the all-over wash easy and a pleasant experience for both of them.

Singing

There is good evidence (Brown et al. 2001) that if staff sing while they work, there is improved posture, eye contact and calmer behaviour in people with dementia. This is a simple and cheap intervention and a consistent finding. It does not matter what staff sing, although there might be greater enjoyment from singing some old songs that are familiar to the person with dementia. It seems that rhythm is very deeply buried in the brain, and even very disabled people with dementia can enjoy and even participate in singing. People who have lost their verbal skills can sometimes sing whole hymns or songs, and will derive huge enjoyment from it. Background music is questionable. In small doses it can be enjoyed, but it needs to be appropriate to the person and not too overwhelming. Turning the television off in care homes is a role that often falls to visiting nurses since the staff have often almost failed to notice that it is on.

Using the arts

Poetry, sculpture, and painting – all are media in which some people with dementia excel, often for the first time in their lives (Basting and Killick 2003). Not all the art is about communication, but some is. Killick (2008) has recorded the words of people with dementia as poetry, and some of it clearly allows the person to share with us what it might be like to be totally bewildered.

With carers

Carers are often older people too, so the usual advice on communication applies. They may also be very tired, angry and frustrated. We professionals fail them so often because we fail to listen properly, we fail to respect what they have to say, and we often fail to be honest about what we can and cannot do (Scenario 6.3). Most carers will say that they really appreciate someone who takes time to listen properly. They do not expect miracles, but they expect respect and recognition. Older carers can be in poor health and very weary. Sons and daughters can be working and bringing up a family and at their wits end. Financial issues can loom large, not just about inheritance but about the actual costs of caring: doing extra washing, cooking, shopping. Of course, we tend to see mostly carers who are struggling.

We have to be careful about making assumptions such as referring to the person with dementia as 'your loved one' since many relationships are not loving but are held together by a sense of duty. Again, listening carefully without making judgements can be very helpful.

Scenario 6.3: Changing relationships

Mr and Mrs Clarke stayed together in late life because the alternative seemed too difficult and too upsetting for their family. They had not enjoyed each other's company for many years, and were living almost separate lives in the same house. When Mr Clarke got dementia, Mrs Clarke felt utterly trapped. She was constantly in a rage with him and with life in general since she was no longer able to do the things that she had enjoyed. She was unable to tell anybody about her feelings and appeared to everyone to be a loyal carer to her husband. She became depressed and was in poor physical health. The district nurse visiting to deal with her leg ulcers never imagined that this was a woman who was desperate to talk properly to someone about her plight.

It can be very demanding for professionals visiting carers, who may be burdened by a variety of emotions such as anxiety, grief, anger or rage, resentment and disappointment. Actively listening and sharing with carers can indeed have a negative impact on the professional's own mental health and ability to help.

Assessment

All the nations of the UK have a policy of single shared assessments to ensure that individuals are not subjected to many different professional assessments, and to enable information to be shared more effectively. The documents and processes vary greatly from one region to another even within the different nations, although the content tends to cover the same subject areas. Such assessments are increasingly electronic, which makes sharing a great deal simpler. Single shared assessments such as the Single Assessment Process (DH 2004) can expose problems between health and social care staff. In most places, local authority assessment staff and all nurses in the community are meant to complete the paperwork, usually on the basis that the person who is first in the door is responsible. Many staff see it as a chore that gets in the way of the real work of helping people, even when they can see the point of thorough information collection and sharing. This is discussed in more detail in Chapter 7.

Ideally, assessments should be joint and shared through members of a team, each contributing their own expertise (Keady et al. 2007). Many such teams exist, especially mental health teams for older people, the most comprehensive of which have staff from both the old age psychiatry service and the local authority. These teams can then agree who is the lead person who will ensure the paperwork is completed and will form the primary link with the family. Many people with dementia will not be the responsibility of an older people's mental health team. They may have been initially referred for diagnosis and treatment, and then referred back to their GP/primary care team for further care.

So where do we start? Many nurses in the community will be working with older people and will have a suspicion that all is not well in the sense that either a relative is saying that the person is becoming very forgetful or there may be incidents such as getting lost, or it may be clear that the person is not coping with daily life. The first step is a visit to the GP to exclude any treatable condition, enabling the GP to diagnose dementia or refer on to a specialist for further investigations, diagnosis and treatment.

Ideally, the person or team who make the diagnosis will share it with the individual and his or her family. Early diagnosis, and sharing of the diagnosis, has many advantages. If appropriate, treatment can be initiated. The person and the family can make adjustments, can access services and can make plans for the future. Many will tell you that it is less frightening to know than to imagine that they are going mad. However, there will be people who prefer not to know, and this must be respected (Iliffe and Manthorpe 2004); people have their own way of coping. Visiting nurses are often called upon to explain the diagnosis more carefully, and this may have to be done several times as the news sinks in. There are many good booklets available through Alzheimer's societies, which can be left to be read when the person and the family are ready. If they are familiar with the Internet, there are many good and reliable sources of information there too.

Having a confirmed diagnosis is therefore step 1 in any assessment. Completing assessment paperwork is best done alongside the people with dementia and their carers so that they can see what is being asked and what is being recorded. Most forms require their signature. This can be a positive experience in helping people to look clearly at their circumstances, and to talk about the issues that arise. Nurses are often in an excellent position to highlight the needs of the person with dementia and his or her carer. By referring on to other professionals for more detailed assessments and interventions, it is often possible to enable the person with dementia to live as normal a life as possible for as long as possible (Scenario 6.4). Community psychiatric nurses and research nurses often use standardised assessment tools when doing a specialist assessment. These include:

- the Mini-Mental State examination (MMSE, Folstein et al. 1975)
- the 6-item Cognitive Impairment Test (6CIT; Brooke and Bullock 1999). The 6CIT is a much newer test than the MMSE, and it would appear to be culturally and linguistically translatable
- the more comprehensive Addenbrooke's Cognitive Examination – Revised (ACE-R; Kipps and Hodges 2008).

Scenario 6.4: Adaptation

Mrs O'Riordan, who had an MMSE score of 9 out of 30, was able to cope living on her own at home because she had a very fixed routine and she used practical skills honed over her lifetime, rather than using cognition.

These need to be used with skill in order to avoid the person with dementia feeling a failure. The tools can give an indication of the type of cognitive impairment but of course do not always provide a picture of competence.

Increasingly, health and social care policy is looking to outcomes, and the assessment and care programmes will have to work towards achieving these. The University of York has worked with older people and their families for a long time and has formulated a set of outcomes based on their views; the University of Glasgow developed these still further. The Joint Improvement Team in Scotland has produced these in an accessible form as part of their User Defined Service Evaluation Toolkit (UDSET) pack (Cook et al. 2007). Assessments should clearly be the first step in working towards these outcomes. For older service users, see Table 6.1.

There is much to think about here. Few single shared assessment forms look at activities or dealing with stigma and discrimination. Few look at the potential for improved confidence and skills. Assessment protocols will probably change as the outcomes approach becomes embedded. In the meantime, there is nothing to stop staff completing assessments from adding these to the paperwork.

Table 6.1 Outcomes important to service users (Cook et al. 2007)

Quality of life	Process	Change
Feeling safe	Being listened to	Improved confidence and skills
Having things to do	Having a say	Improved mobility
Seeing people	Being treated with respect	Reduced symptoms
Staying as well as you can be	Being treated as an individual	
Living where you want/as you want	Responsiveness	
Dealing with stigma/discrimination	Reliability	

Working with carers

Although communication with carers was mentioned above, it may be helpful to have a specific section of this chapter on working with carers. Their key role can be overlooked, and there is strong evidence that working intensively with carers can enable them to cope for a longer period (Mittelman 1997). A good place to start is outcomes identified from the UDSET pack (Cook et al. 2007). A separate carer assessment is now a statutory requirement (although there is no statutory requirement to provide services) in all parts of the UK, and these documents too will shift to more of an outcome focus. Table 6.2 gives much food for thought and presents many challenges to staff visiting carers at home.

Although some of it is well accepted, we often fail to appreciate the importance of managing the caring role. Do carers have choices? Can they tell us the limits of what they feel able to do? Are they sufficiently informed, skilled and equipped? There is now very good research evidence (Brodarty et al. 2003) that carer training can be really effective. Satisfaction in caring is something where we can really help. We can offer respect, encouragement and positive regard, which may be in short supply. If we feel a good job is being done, we should say so. We should see ourselves as partners in the caring role for some people, and it is clear from Table 6.2 that this is what carers would like. They are not our partners, we are theirs – a subtle difference that highlights where the control should lie. The processes carers consider important seem obvious but are really difficult to achieve. Some are about our attitudes and the way we relate to them. Being flexible and responsive to changing needs is really challenging and particularly important in dementia care, where any change

Table 6.2 Outcomes important to carers (Cook et al. 2007)

Quality of life for the cared for person	Quality of life for the carer	Managing the caring role	Process
Quality of life for the cared for person	Maintaining health and well-being A life of their own Positive relationship with the person cared for Freedom from financial hardship	Choices in caring, including the limits of caring Feeling informed/ skilled/equipped Satisfaction in caring Partnership with services	Valued/respected and expertise recognised Having a say in services Flexible and responsive to changing needs Positive/meaningful relationship with practitioners Accessible, available and free at the point of need

can have profound implications. If a few hours extra help is not available when there is a crisis, such as a carer falling ill, a really negative sequence of events may follow.

Working with other agencies and professionals

The 'assessment' section above alluded to some problems between agencies, which will be spelled out here. In my view, there is no use pretending that the medical and social approaches are similar and can be integrated. It is much more useful to see them both as essential – two sides of the same coin perhaps. Nurses in the community fall, often painfully, between them. They are comfortable with a medical view and a focus on clinical treatment, yet they know a lot about social factors, which are affecting the people with whom they work.

It is also not useful to pretend that there is rarely a power struggle going on between social and health organisations. There are very few resources in the community, and agencies will try hard to shift costs to other agencies. All UK governments have tried really hard to promote collaboration and joint working, and have made considerable progress in this area, but many tensions remain. At community level, staff often get on very well. If they know and like each other, they share responsibility to get the best deal possible from the resources available. Many teams work well, as do many networks, especially between nurses and social workers.

The key to collaboration is being confident in your own skills and able to cope with the overlap with other professions. Some people manage this better than others. Some people, perhaps those who are less secure in their professional role, stick to it rigidly and project much of their frustration elsewhere. The lives and needs of people with dementia are so complicated that only people willing to be flexible and creative can really deliver services of real quality. Those who do work well together generally:

- know each other well, and will provide support and encouragement as well as appreciation to each other
- know about the roles of colleagues: what can they offer, what is not possible, what approach they take, what priorities they have to meet
- are open to discussing difficulties and learn from one another
- know how to access services from other agencies – as one mentor used to say, 'You are only as good as your contacts'
- know what is available in the community.

The most important agency is probably the local Alzheimer's Society, which can offer a range of services such as day care, befriending and, most importantly, information. Voluntary organisations change very quickly as they obtain and lose funding so it is crucial to check regularly what is on offer. Usually, a new service takes a while to settle so you can get the best if you can get in quickly. Other voluntary organisations offer all sorts of services: advocacy, respite at home, clubs, activities such as art or drama and holidays. There is no possibility of listing what is available because it varies so greatly from place to place.

The way services are run also varies enormously, and new kinds of service keep appearing too. Alzheimer cafés, for example, are regular social gatherings, perhaps one evening a month, for people with dementia and their carers. There is usually food and drink, which makes it an evening out, and usually a talk from a professional. Alzheimer Society of Ireland has started a new sort of club, which seems to be working very well. These clubs are for people with dementia and their relatives. Refreshments are served (usually lots of tea), but what happens depends on the participants who run the club; the staff of the Society simply do the basic organisation. Being in control or having a say was identified in Table 6.2 as being important for carers. Both these services demonstrate an increasing recognition that many people with dementia and their carers like to socialise together, and that this can be difficult because the person with dementia may no longer be able to cope with normal social occasions.

Technology

This issue is given a subsection because it is emerging as a crucial part of care packages (Woolham 2005), yet there may be some anxiety about its purpose. Devices can be helpful and should be a way of demonstrating that technology ought to be an integral part of our thinking. It does not replace one-to-one contacts, but it can provide additional help especially to people who live on their own. Technology is anything from a maxiplug that opens when the bath gets too full, to a monitoring system linked to a community alarm service computer. Some devices, such as those which use a taped message linked to front door magnets, to advise the person with dementia not to go out because it is during the night, are not only helpful to the person with dementia, but also a comfort to the carers. Movement detectors are now available in most DIY stores so carers can install them themselves. They can, for example, be linked to the hall light so that the person with dementia can find their way to the toilet when they get up at night. We discuss some further examples of technology in Chapter 7.

Challenges and rewards

Minority ethnic groups

It feels awkward putting minority ethnic groups into a section on challenges and rewards when working with people from minority ethnic groups is increasingly mainstream. The NAO report (2007) says there are about 15,000 people from minority communities with dementia and that this will rise sharply with increasing numbers of older people. But the reality is that many community staff are anxious about how to proceed, and many non-indigenous people with dementia fail to receive a good service. The first step is to be aware that dementia may be understood differently by different cultures. A sound person-centred approach is the way to proceed: make no assumptions and listen carefully. An interpreter may be needed, and it may be necessary to find out how they themselves view dementia, to ensure that they too are really listening. Most research indicates that people born in other countries want the same as those born in the UK (Patel 2004), but services do need to be culturally sensitive (Scenario 6.5).

Scenario 6.5: Culture

Staff in two day centres in Edinburgh were given intensive training in culturally sensitive behaviour because there was no possibility of separate day care for the small number of people from different cultures using them. The results were very clear: appreciative users and increasing use by ethnic minority groups.

It is not just people with dementia who may come from other countries – it may also be staff. Indeed you, the reader, may have migrated to the UK. You may well be struggling with communication issues and the attitudes of people with dementia. They may have attitudes shaped many years ago. Intensive training of the staff from overseas may be required to ensure they understand more about the people they are caring for.

Behaviour

The behaviour of people with dementia can sometimes be problematic to them, their carers and staff (Chapman et al. 2007). The causes of challenging behaviour can be multiple. Occasionally, they may be directly related to brain damage, and it can be helpful to know what type of dementia the person has; however, it is always a good idea to work on the assumption that behaviour is an attempt to communicate and then to work back to a more pathological explanation as a last resort. A helpful approach is the detective one (James et al. 2006): assuming that the person is attempting to communicate something and to work out what that is and why they are using that particular behaviour. The NICE/SCIE guidelines (2006) have an excellent section on non-cognitive problems in dementia, and they describe this process more formally in terms of lists of possibilities to assess. The first step is to describe the behaviour carefully and to see what sparks it off (Stokes 2001) (Scenario 6.6).

Scenario 6.6: Behaviour 1

Mr Johnson is referred because he is a 'wanderer'. He is always trying to get out of the house, which places great strain on his disabled wife who cannot go with him or after him. You discover from his past life that he has always been a great walker. He walked to work and he walked in the hills at the weekend. He cannot understand why his wife tries to prevent him going out walking now, because he cannot remember that he gets lost. This is creating nearly intolerable frustration and tension in this household. The answer may be to find an organisation that offers befriending so someone can walk with him. In the near future, he will be able to use GPS technology, although if he gets lost Mrs Johnson will need help to bring him home.

Some people with dementia are described as 'aggressive' or 'resistant', yet when the behaviour is carefully described, it can be clear that this is often when they are being helped with intimate care. Perhaps it is painful. Pain is too often not considered or treated in people with dementia (McClean and Cunningham 2007). Perhaps it reminds them of some trauma such as sexual abuse in the past. Carers may need help to think carefully about this and to work out a plan to try various changes in routine to see if they help.

Mr Johnson's story is straightforward, but some are more complicated. Angry behaviour often relates to frustration at diminishing competence. People can understandably be angry and lash out. The answer may be to assess remaining competence and organise tasks to take advantage of this.

Some people become more disinhibited and use foul language or are sexually more demanding. The extent to which this is a problem depends on the relationship and attitudes of the carer or care home staff. Skilled counselling may be required from the visiting nurse. The old adage that older people often want to talk about sex and death but we professionals are not brave enough is useful to bear in mind.

Much behaviour is an attempt to communicate boredom and feelings of uselessness. Carers and care home staff may need help in working out ways to help people with dementia pass the time and feel useful (Scenario 6.7). Creative thinking is really essential in dementia care, as are activities (Knocker 2003).

Scenario 6.7: Behaviour 2

Mr Porter, a retired plumber, was angry when he was prevented from dismantling the central heating radiators in his care home. When he was given a toolbox full of tools and bits of pipework, he was absorbed for hours in sorting it all out.

Carers and care home staff may need to be encouraged to find ways of involving the person with dementia, because there is always a tendency to do a job yourself, which is quicker and easier. Maintaining past hobbies is often a challenge, and having good friends who will take the person with dementia to bowls or to the pub can be really helpful. Carers can be so tired and overwhelmed that they need help in seeing that there may be a constructive solution if the behaviour is seen as communication (Scenario 6.8).

Scenario 6.8: Behaviour 3

Mrs Cuthbertson was very disabled with her dementia, but she really enjoyed going through piles of lentils, picking out the discoloured ones. Her husband would then make lentil soup and was able to express his appreciation for her efforts.

There will of course be occasions when drastic action is called for, and the use of neuroleptics is indicated. This should always be a last resort, and if they are used, a record must be kept which not only describes the behaviour but indicates when the medication will be reviewed. These drugs have a relatively short period of effectiveness, so should not be used in the long term. They also have side-effects, not least impairing the competence and confidence of the person with dementia. Issues of covert medication and dementia are usually related to these drugs. A Nursing and Midwifery Council (2007) guideline exists for this. There are good guidelines for the care of people with dementia with behaviour problems and the use of neuroleptics in the NICE/SCIE (2006) report.

Abuse

Older people with dementia are often abused and often abuse (Scenario 6.9).

Scenario 6.9: Abuse 1

Mr MacKay was very angry and frustrated with his dementia and often hit his wife with his walking stick. She understood why he was doing it, but she was increasingly afraid.

Reflection points

● **What would you do if you were visiting Mr and Mrs Mackay?**

Abuse can take many forms: neglect, financial abuse, physical abuse, sexual abuse and so on. It can take place at home and in care homes, and it can be perpetrated by relatives and by staff and even by strangers (Scenario 6.10).

Scenario 6.10: Abuse 2

Mrs Emmerson was visited regularly by a couple of strangers who asked her for money, which she gave them. She appeared to be both grateful for their company and sorry for them. Her daughter had to take charge of her finances to stop this happening.

The Alzheimer's Society in conjunction with Action on Elder Abuse has published a useful book (2008) about abuse in care homes and what to do if you suspect it is going on. There is really good literature on abuse and older people, much of it by Pritchard (2008). In each of the countries of the UK, there is now new legislation about the protection of vulnerable adults. The NICE/SCIE guidelines (2006) recommend:

Because people with dementia are vulnerable to abuse and neglect, all health and social care staff should receive information and training about, and abide by the local multi-agency policy on, adult protection. (p. 15)

Polypharmacy

Many people with dementia, like older people generally, are at risk of polypharmacy. They may be on repeat prescriptions, their medication may not have been reviewed, they may have medication from the hospital and from their GP practice, and they may be using over-the-counter medication or alternative therapies as well as prescribed medication. The results can be really serious, even fatal. Competence can be seriously diminished and health impaired. Nurses have a lot of skill and knowledge related to medication issues and are the key professionals in the community to take action. A medication review is essential. Once it is clear what is being taken, an assessment of concordance is the first step. Once this has happened, there may need to be arrangements to assist with concordance. In some places, home care staff are trained to give medication; in others they are allowed to remind people. Some people with dementia can manage with a daily dose reminder or a monitored dosage system, although there is little research looking at their effectiveness. Nurses may also have a key role in advising staff in care homes about medication and when it would be useful to seek a review from the GP.

Sleep

Not getting enough sleep is a problem for both people with dementia and their carers and can lie behind a lot of problems (Bephage 2007). Yet if it is carefully investigated, there are often ways of helping (Scenario 6.11).

Scenario 6.11: Sleep solution

Miss Thomas was lying awake to pre-empt her father with dementia from getting up in the night and going downstairs or outside, or to help him find his way to the toilet. She found a passive infrared detector across the top of the stairs linked to a bell in her bedroom useful. She also installed a low light on a plug, which remained permanently on to make sure the way to the bathroom was visible.

There are many possible solutions to sleep disturbance. The person with dementia may no longer be able to judge the time, in which case a large, clear clock with a low light permanently on it may help. The person with dementia may not find it easy to get off to sleep, perhaps because they have had no exercise during the day or because they have lost their pre-bed routine. This can be reinstated with a quiet period before bed, perhaps some warm milk and honey, or whatever was their routine in the past.

Sundowning is a term for a period of restlessness that seems to occur in some people with dementia in the early evening. There are many possible explanations, such as the possibility that this is the time people used to leave work or welcome their husbands from work, or it may be the result of the shift change in the care home. It can be problematic for staff, and they may need help ensuring that the routines in the care home aim for a calm and quiet period at this time, ideally with some extra staff.

Food and drink

People with dementia who live alone raise a lot of concern about their ability to get enough food and drink (Marshall 2003a, 2003b; Alzheimer's Society 2004). They may no longer be able to shop but rely on Meals on Wheels, which can be baffling: the foil trays make no sense and the microwave is a mystery. People with dementia can lose their cooking skills. A careful assessment is needed to check if they ever had any or what they retain, and to judge how important cooking is to them (Wey 2005). Sometimes they only need one of the burners on the stove to heat up tinned beans; sometimes they are keen to cook a proper meal. Automatically assuming they are going to set the house or flat on fire is not helpful since removing the stove often precipitates a rapid drop in independence. Technology can help in making cookers safer. Induction cookers are one option for the financially better off since they only heat what is in the pan and go off when there is no liquid left. Another option is a heat detector, which switches the cooker off if it gets too hot.

Ensuring people with dementia get enough to drink is a challenge. Poor hydration is implicated in many health problems, such as constipation, falls, delirium and urinary tract infections (Archibald 2005). People who are in their 80s today rarely drank glasses of water except with meals; they drank tea, yet they may no longer be able to work the kettle, especially if it is a very modern one. Lots of ready-made juices in easy to understand jugs will be the answer for some people. For others, it may be about informing friends and neighbours about the importance of hydration so that they can offer a familiar drink. They may be unwilling to do this in the evening because of fears of a wet bed. Again, they may need to be told about the risk of constipation and urinary tract infection with too little liquid. Special efforts may need to be made to make the journey to the toilet in the night a safe one with extra lighting.

Food and drink are just as much a problem in residential and nursing homes (Berg 2006). One possibility is to convert a little used lounge into a café. People with dementia know how to behave in a café, and they eat and drink without thinking about it. Nurses will find themselves constantly reminding carers and care staff that people with dementia often cannot remember to eat and drink, so food and drink need to be visible and in acceptable and understandable forms. Some cannot even remember how to eat or use cutlery, so eating alongside them can be very helpful. It is worth remembering that poor nutrition has an effect on both physical and mental health.

Reflection points

- Why do you think nurses are not getting involved in food and drink issues as much as they used to?

Food and drink problems tax the imagination of all professionals involved, because the answer depends on knowing about the individuals, their competence, their habits and their routines.

End of life care

This has been a neglected issue for a long time, but more material is now available (Downs et al. 2006). Many issues arise about intensive treatment and resuscitation, which are much easier to deal with if there has been a full discussion when the person with dementia was able to voice an opinion. Some people with dementia clearly have a really good quality of life; so a diagnosis is not, in itself, guidance on the best course of action.

Most people with dementia do not die in their own homes or even in care homes – they die in hospitals – however, with support, dying at home or in a care home can be made more possible. Hudson (2003) has good suggestions about better palliative care in care homes. The special problems for people with dementia and their carers often relate to pain assessment when the person with dementia is unable to provide verbal information. Carers and professionals have to rely on non-verbal cues, which can cause high levels of anxiety.

Grief is a very personal business; some carers may well have grieved enough along the journey, whereas others will be overwhelmed at the actual death of the person with dementia. Bereaved carers of people with dementia may be particularly tired and vulnerable, and may welcome a lot of support.

Not enough time

Every part of this chapter has emphasised the need to take time. People with dementia need time. Their thought processes can be slower. They can be slower to get accustomed to a visitor and to trust them. It often takes time to really get to know them and their history, preferences, etc. Yet this is not often sufficiently understood by managers who decide how much work a nurse in the community can achieve.

Consistency

At the start of this chapter, we discussed the fact that professionals are seldom able to journey for any length of time with a person with dementia and their carer. Yet when asked, many carers and people with dementia say that they greatly value a consistent person and find a traffic of strangers very unhelpful. One woman said her home was like a railway station. Another had 26 different people calling in one week. If you have an impaired memory and a limited grasp on what is going on, this is profoundly unsatisfactory.

Looking after yourself

Working with people with dementia and their carers in the community is not easy and can indeed be very stressful (Sammut 2003a, Sammut 2003b). Staff rarely have enough time to do it well and to feel satisfied with their intervention. They get involved with many sad situations with distressed and angry carers and vulnerable and stressed people with dementia. It is really important to attend to the impact of this work and to seek support. This may take the form of colleague support, perhaps a regular group for sharing of problems. Regular debriefing or clinical supervision is really crucial if we are to retain our imagination and empathy in the field. This is not regularly offered to nurses but it should be. It is too easy to lapse into task-centred work, we do the basic job but attend to nothing else. Sometimes it is the employing organisation which is the problem. There can be a lack of staff support, a large number sick colleagues or unfilled vacancies. Unwinding at the end of the day is important and should be taken seriously, as should the signs of real stress such as poor sleeping, loss of empathy, a short temper and an inability to concentrate.

Humour

People with dementia do not necessarily lose their sense of humour, nor do carers, although the daily worries may not make this evident. Humour can be a great release of tension (Scenario 6.12).

Scenario 6.12: Humour

Mrs de Rollo claimed there was a third person in her marriage called Mr Alzheimer, who kept making her do ridiculous things. She and her husband used *him* as a way of laughing about their situation with her dementia.

Finding opportunities for shared laughter such as DVDs of old television series can be very therapeutic. Carers are often embarrassed to laugh about some of the unlikely things that happen as a result of dementia. You may need to laugh with them as long as it is kindly meant. Carers' groups can laugh a lot at shared anecdotes and can feel better as a consequence.

Rewards

Most textbooks about working with people with dementia focus on the problems and ignore the rewards. There is an overemphasis on carer stress and burden when we know that it is not the majority who feel stressed (although, as professionals, these do tend to be the people we see). We may need to stop and consider the rewards of this work. These can include getting to know people who are facing one of life's greatest challenges with courage and dignity. Feeling that we have done something to help make the journey less painful by *travelling* with the person with dementia is reward in itself.

Conclusion

Nurses can make a difference to people with dementia, who can learn new things, take part in the rehabilitation process and have a quality of life never anticipated. Dementia care is a very dynamic field with new approaches being established all the time. It is a field of work that suits creative people who are willing to think out of the box to solve what can be very complicated problems. There are a large number of wonderful professionals in dementia care, and working with them is one of the great rewards of this field. Many people like a challenge in their work and gain rewards from doing it well.

Acknowledgements

Special thanks are due to Gillian Irvine, Angela Hudson and Gillian Boardman, who provided much useful commentary.

References

Adams, T. (2001) The social construction of risk by community psychiatric nurses and family carers for people with dementia. *Health Risk and Society* 3(3): 307–20.

Adams, T. (2008) Nursing people with dementia and their family members – towards a whole systems approach. In T. Adams (ed.) (2008) *Dementia Care Nursing, Promoting Well Being in People with Dementia and their Families.* Basingstoke: Palgrave Macmillan.

Allan, K. (2001) *Communication and Consultation: Exploring Ways for Staff to Involve People with Dementia in Developing Services.* Bristol: Policy Press.

Alzheimer's Society and Action on Elder Abuse (2008) *Uncovering Abuse in the Dementia Care Environment.* London: Alzheimer's Society.

Alzheimer's Society (2001) *Quality Dementia Care in Care Homes: Person Centred Standards.* London: Alzheimer's Society.

Alzheimer's Society (2004) *Food for Thought. Promoting Quality: Food and Nutrition for people with Dementia, Practice Guides.* London: Alzheimer's Society.

Alzheimer's Society (2007*) Dementia UK.* London: Alzheimer's Society.

Anderson, E. (2008) Cognitive change in old age. In R. Jacoby, C. Oppenheimer, T. Dening and A. Thomas (eds.) *Oxford Textbook of Old Age Psychiatry.* Oxford: Oxford University Press.

Archibald, C. (2005) *Rehydration and Dementia.* Stirling: Dementia Services Development Centre.

Audit Commission (2000) *Forget Me Not: Older People with Mental Health Problems.* Available from http://www.audit-commission.gov.uk/reports/.

Audit Commission (2002) *Forget Me Not 2002: Developing Mental Health Services for Older People in England.* Available from http://www.audit-commission.gov.uk/reports/.

Basting, A.D. and Killick, J. (2003) *The Arts and Dementia Care, a Resources Guide.* New York: Centre for Creative Ageing.

Bender, M. (2004) *Therapeutic Group Work for People with Cognitive Losses: Working with People with Dementia.* Bicester: Speechmark.

Bephage, G. (2007) Care approaches to sleeplessness and dementia. *Nursing and Residential Care* 9(12): 571–3.

Berg, G. (2006) *The Importance of Food and Mealtimes in Dementia Care.* London: Jessica Kingsley.

Brodarty, H., Green, A. and Koschera, A. (2003) Meta-analysis of psychosocial interventions for caregivers of people with dementia. *Journal of the American Geriatric Society* 51(5): 657–64.

Brooke, P. and Bullock, R. (1999) Validation of the 6 item cognitive impairment test. *International Journal of Geriatric Psychiatry* 14: 936–40.

Brooker, D. (2008) Person centred care. In R. Jacoby, C. Oppenheimer, T. Dening and A. Thomas (eds.) *Oxford Textbook of Old Age Psychiatry.* Oxford: Oxford University Press.

Brooker, D. and Woolley, R. (2006) Enriched activity programme for people with dementia: the development and evaluation of a new model for working with people with dementia. Available from http://www.brad.ac.uk/health/dementia/research/enriched.php.

Brown, S., Gotell, E. and Ekman, S.L. (2001) Singing as an intervention in dementia care. *Journal of Dementia Care* 9(4): 33–7.

Bryans, M., Keady, J., Turner, S., Wilcock, J., Downs, M. and Iliffe, S. (2003) An exploratory survey into primary care nurses and dementia care. *British Journal of Nursing* 12(17): 1029–37.

Bryden, C. (2005) *Dancing with Dementia.* London: Jessica Kingsley.

Care Services Improvement Partnership (2005) *Everybody's Business: Integrated Services for Older Adults: A Service Development Guide.* London: HMSO.

Chapman, A., Jackson, G. and MacDonald, C. (2007) *What behaviour? Whose Problem?* Stirling: Dementia Services Development Centre.

Cheston, R., Jones, K. and Gilliard, J. (2003) Group psychotherapy and people with dementia. *Ageing and Mental Health* 7(6): 452–61.

Clare, L. (2005) Cognitive rehabilitation for people with dementia. In M. Marshall (ed.) *Perspectives on Rehabilitation and Dementia.* London: Jessica Kingsley.

Cook, A., Miller, E. and Whorisky, M. (2007) *Do Health and Social Care Partnerships Deliver Good Outcomes to Service users and Carers? Development of the User Defined Service Evaluation Toolkit (UDSET).* Available from www.jitscotland.org.uk.

Crisp, J. (2003) Communication. In R. Hudson (ed.) *Dementia Nursing: A Guide to Practice.* Melbourne: Ausmed Publications.

Cunningham, C., Kerr, D. and McClean, W. (2007) *Differential Diagnosis Tool: Identifying possible Causes of Changes that Mimic Dementia.* Stirling: Dementia Services Development Centre.

Department of Health (2001) *The National Service Framework for Older People*. Available from http://www.dh.gov.uk/en/Publicationsandstatistics/Publications/PublicationsPolicyAndGuidance/DH_4003066.

Department of Health (2004) *Single Assessment Process Implementation (SAP) Guidance*, Available from http://www.dh.gov.uk/en/SocialCare/Chargingandassessment/SingleAssessmentProcess/index.htm.

Department of Health (2008) *National Dementia Strategy*. Available from http://www.dh.gov.uk/en/SocialCare/Deliveringadultsocialcare/Olderpeople/NationalDementiaStrategy/index.htm.

Dewing, J. and Blackburn, S. (1999) Dementia, part 4: risk assessment. *Professional Nurse* 14(11): 803–5.

Downs, M., Small, N. and Froggatt, N. (2006) Explanatory models of dementia: links to end-of-life care. *International Journal of Palliative Nursing* 12(5): 209–13.

Folstein, M.F., Folstein, S.E. and McHugh, P.R. (1975) Mini-Mental State: a practical method for grading the cognitive state of patients for the clinician. *Journal of Psychiatric Research* 12: 189–198.

Frataglioni, L., von Strauss, E. and Qui, C. (2008) Epidemiology of the dementias of old age. In R. Jacoby, C. Oppenheimer, T. Dening and A. Thomas (eds.) *Oxford Textbook of Old Age Psychiatry*. Oxford: Oxford University Press.

Gilmour, H. (2004) Living alone with dementia: risk and the professional role. *Nursing Older People* 16(9): 20–5.

Goldsmith, M. (2004) *Ageing in a Strange Land: People with Dementia and the Local Church*. Edinburgh: 4M Publications.

Hogg, J. (2008) Delirium. In R. Jacoby, C. Oppenheimer, T. Dening and A. Thomas (eds.) *Oxford Textbook of Old Age Psychiatry*. Oxford University Press: Oxford.

Holmes, C. (2008) The genetics and molecular biology of dementia. In R. Jacoby, C. Oppenheimer, T. Dening and A. Thomas (eds.) *Oxford Textbook of Old Age Psychiatry*. Oxford University Press: Oxford.

Hudson, R. (2003) *Dementia Nursing: A guide to practice*. Melbourne: Ausmed Publications.

Huusko, T.M., Karppi, P., Avikainen, V., Kautiainen, K. and Sulkava, R. (2000) Randomised, clinically controlled trial of intensive geriatric rehabilitation in patients with hip fracture: subgroup analysis of patients with dementia. *BMJ* 321: 1107–11.

Illife, S. and Manthorpe, J. (2004) The hazards of early recognition of dementia: a risk assessment. *Aging and Mental Health* 8(2): 99–105.

Innes, A., Archibald, C. and Murphy, C. (2004) *Dementia and Social Inclusion. Marginalised Groups and Marginalised Areas of Dementia Research, Care and Practice*. London: Jessica Kingsley Publishers.

James, I., Mackenzie, L., Stephenson, M. and Roe, T. (2006) Dealing with challenging behaviour through an analysis of need: the Colombo approach. In M. Marshall and K. Allan eds.) *Dementia: Walking not Wandering*. London: Hawker Publications.

Keady, J., Clarke, C. and Page, S. (2007) *Partnerships in Community Mental Health Nursing and Dementia Care: Practice and Perspectives*. Buckingham: Open University Press.

Killick, J. (2008) *Dementia Diary: Poems and Prose*. London: Hawker Publications.

Kipps, C.M. and Hodges, J. (2008) Clinical cognitive assessment. In R. Jacoby, C. Oppenheimer, T. Dening and A. Thomas (eds.) (2008) *Oxford Textbook of Old Age Psychiatry*. Oxford: Oxford University Press.

Kitwood, T. (1997) *Dementia Reconsidered: The Person Comes First*. Buckingham: Open University Press.

Knocker, S. (2003) *Alzheimer's Society Book of Activities*. London: Alzheimer's Society.

McAndrew, F. and Taylor, R. (2006) How all voices are heard for strategic planning. *Journal of Dementia Care* 14(3): 22–4.

McLean, W. and Cunningham, C. (2007) *Pain in Older People and People with Dementia: A Practice Guide*. Stirling: Dementia Services Development Centre.

Manning, W. (2003) *Delirium*. Stirling: Dementia Services Development Centre.

Manthorpe, J. (2003) Risk and dementia: models for community mental health nursing practice. In J. Keady, C. Clarke and T. Adams (eds.) (2003) *Community Mental Health Nursing and Dementia Care: Practice Perspectives*. Buckingham: Open University Press.

Manthorpe, J. and Illiffe, S. (2005) *Depression in Later Life*. London: Jessica Kingsley.

Manthorpe, J. and Illiffe, S. (2007) Timely recognition of dementia: community nurses crucial roles. *British Journal of Community Nursing* 12(2): 74–6.

Marshall, M. (ed.) (2003a) *Food, Glorious Food: Perspectives on Food and Dementia*. London: Hawker Publications.

Marshall, M. (2003b) Nutrition. In Hudson, R. (ed.) (2003) *Dementia Nursing: A Guide to Practice*. Melbourne: Ausmed Publications.

Marshall, M. (2005) *Perspectives on Rehabilitation and Dementia*. London: Jessica Kingsley.

Marshall, M. and Allan, K. (eds.) (2006) *Dementia: Walking not Wandering. Fresh Approaches to Understanding and Practice*. London: Hawker Publications.

Mittelman, M.S., Ferris, S.H., Shulman, E., Steinberg, G., Ambinder, A. and Mackell, J. (1997) The effects of a multi component support program on spouse-caregivers of Alzheimer's disease patients: results of a treatment/control study. In Heston, L.L. (ed.) (1997) *Progress in Alzheimer's disease and Similar Conditions*. Washington, DC: American Psychiatric Press.

Nagy, Z. and Hubbard, P. (2008) Neuropathology. In Jacoby, R., Oppenheimer, C., Dening, T. and Thomas, A. (eds.) (2008) *Oxford Textbook of Old Age Psychiatry*. Oxford: Oxford University Press.

National Audit Office (2007) *Improving Services and Support for People with Dementia*. Available from http://www.official-documents.gov.uk/document/hc0607/hc06/0604/0604.asp.

National Institute for Health and Clinical Excellence (2007) *Alzheimer's Disease – Donepezil, Galantamine, Rivastigmine (Review) and Memantine. Technology Appraisal*. NICE: London, available from http://www.nice.org.uk/TA111.

National Institute for Health and Clinical Excellence and Social Care Institute for Excellence (2006) *Dementia: Supporting People with Dementia and their Carers in Health and Social Care.* Available from http://www.nice.org.uk/nicemedia/pdf/CG042NICEGuideline.pdf#null.

Nolan, M. (2004) Beyond person centred care: a new vision for gerontological nursing? *International Journal of Older People Nursing* 13(3a): 45–53.

Nolan, M.R., Brown, J., Davies, S., Keady, J. and Nolan, J. (2002) *Longitudinal Study of the Effectiveness of Educational Preparation to Meet the Needs of Older People and their Carers: The Advancing Gerontological Education in Nursing (The AGEIN) Project.* ENB Research Highlights No. 48. London: English National Board for Nursing, Midwifery and Health Visiting.

Nolan, M., Davies, S., Ryan, T. and Keady, J. (2008) Relationship-centred care and the 'senses framework'. *Journal of Dementia Care* 16(1): 26–8.

Norman, H.K., Asplund, K., Karlesson, S., Sandman, P.O. and Norberg, A. (2006) People with severe dementia exhibit episodes of lucidity: a population-based study. *Journal of Clinical Nursing* 15(11):1413–17.

Nursing and Midwifery Council (2007) *Covert Administration of Medicines – Disguising Medicine in Food and Drink.* Available from http://www.nmc-uk.org/aFrameDisplay.aspx?DocumentID=4007&Keyword=.

Nursing and Midwifery Council (2008) *Standards of Conduct, Performance and Ethics for Nurses and Midwives.* Available from http://www.nmc-uk.org/aArticle.aspx?ArticleID=3057.

O'Connell, H. and Lawler, B. (2008) Alcohol and substance abuse in older people. In Jacoby, R., Oppenheimer, C., Dening, T. and Thomas, A. (eds.) (2008) *Oxford Textbook of Old Age Psychiatry.* Oxford: Oxford University Press.

Olin, J.T., Katz, I.R., Meyers, B.S., Shneider, L.S. and Lebowitz, B.D. (2002) Provisional diagnostic criteria for depression of Alzheimer's disease: rationale and background. *American Journal of Geriatric Psychiatry* 10(2): 129–141.

Patel, N. (ed.) (2004) *Minority Elderly Health and Social Care in Europe: PRIAE Research briefing. Summary Findings of the Minority Elderly Care (MEC) Project.* Available from http://www.priae.org/.

Post, S.G. (2000) The concept of Alzheimer disease in a hypercognitive society. In Whitehouse, P.J., Maurer, K. and Ballenger, J.F. (eds.) (2000) *Concepts of Alzheimer's Disease. Biological, Clinical and Cultural Perspectives.* Baltimore: Johns Hopkins University Press.

Pritchard, J. (2008) *Good Practice in Safeguarding Adults.* London: Jessica Kingsley Publishers.

Robinson, L., Clare, L. and Evans, K. (2005) Making sense of dementia and adjusting to loss: psychological reactions to a diagnosis of dementia in couples. *Ageing and Mental Health* 9(4): 337–47.

Sammut, A. (2003a) Developing an Appropriate Response to Emotional Pain, *Journal of Dementia Care* 11(2): 23–25.

Sammut, A. (2003b) What about me? Support for dementia care staff. *Journal of Dementia Care* 11(6): 22–4.

Stokes, G. (2001) *Challenging Behaviour in Dementia: A Person-Centred Approach.* Bicester: Speechmark.

Thom, K.M. and Blair, S.E. (1998) Risk in dementia – assessment and management: a literature review. *British Journal of Occupational Therapy* 61: 441–7.

Titterton, M. (2004) *Risk and Risk Taking in Health and Social Welfare*. London: Jessica Kingsley.

Wey, S. (2005) One size does not fit all: person-centred approaches to the use of assistive technology. In M. Marshall (ed.) (2005) *Perspectives on Rehabilitation and Dementia*. London: Jessica Kingsley.

World Health Organization (1990) International Classification of Diseases 10th Revision. Available from http://www.who.int/classifications/icd/en/.

Woolham, J. (ed.) (2005) *Developing the Role of Technology in the Care and Rehabilitation of People with Dementia – Current Trends and Perspectives*. London: Hawker Publications.

Useful websites

Alzheimer's Society: http://www.alzheimers.org.uk

Alzheimer's Society leaflets: http://www.alzheimers.org.uk/site/scripts/documents. php?categoryID=200120)

British Medical Journal: http://besthealth.bmj.com/btuk/conditions/10100.html

Section 3
Future challenges

Chapter 7
Future trends

Lesley Moore and Angela Hudson

Introduction

This chapter is perhaps the most challenging to write as we are looking towards the future, which is rapidly evolving. In our research for this chapter, we have travelled to many parts of the UK to explore some future trends enabled by early adopters of information technology (IT) projects and a genuine attempt to work towards a 'seamless' care system, and one that promotes and supports as far possible the autonomy of the patient. In trying to connect and sense the future that this new century will bring for the care of the older person in the community, we have, as Scharmer (2007) advises, tried to keep an 'open mind', an 'open heart' and an 'open will' so that we can learn. We are a part of that future and its construct, and we owe it to the older people of today and the future to take time to reflect and make sense of the rapid change, and to share our thoughts and concerns. Scharmer (2007) has coined the term 'presencing', which is a blend of the two words 'presence' and 'sensing' and means: 'to sense, tune in, and act from one's highest potential – the future that depends on us to bring it into being' (p. 8).

The being of a new National Health Service (NHS) and social care will be our construct in an age when the user's voice will contribute to decision-making. It has already commenced, and we hope to share some of the founding initiatives that hopefully will underpin the infrastructure of a caring society. Therefore this chapter will explore significant trends leading to the 60th year of the NHS and beyond; the empowerment of the patient through the Expert Patients Programme; the National Programme of IT; the Supporting People initiative; telemedicine, telenursing, telehealth, telecare and e-health. These are but a few of the dimensions of the bigger picture of a future NHS evolving. As Darzi (2008: 15) states, 'it is relatively easy to set out a vision, much harder to make it a reality'. It will need clear leadership and a commitment to change and partnership working across various agencies.

Significant trends leading to the 60th year of the NHS

Within the first decade of the 21st century, we have celebrated the 60th anniversary of the NHS and witnessed the growth and advancement of IT and staff development, and changes in how healthcare is accessed and delivered. The picture of today's healthcare is vastly different from that at its inception, when the UK was still recovering from the devastation of the Second World War, and health and social care agencies were struggling to meet the needs of the wounded military personnel and the dependents of those who did not return from the war. As Green (2008) reflected, many hospitals were under the control of local councils and originated from workhouses. Modern medicines such as antibiotics that we now take for granted were just being discovered and being made available. As Chapman (2008: 19) identified 'there was an influx of people needing treatment of long-standing conditions that had been left untreated', and for many this often meant an early death due to, for example, tuberculosis and bronchitis.

Since its inception, the NHS has grown immensely and has for some time been struggling to meet the health-need demands and the wants of the nation. Technology has produced a vast range of antibiotics that, sadly, are rarely effective today owing to the growth of resistant strains of bacteria. This has led to some devastating consequences for the populace living with long-term conditions (LTCs) such as chronic obstructive pulmonary disease (COPD), and the older person exposed to nosocomial infections such as *Clostridium difficile*, while being cared for in healthcare settings. Although antibiotics made a considerable difference to the control of tuberculosis in the UK in the early 1950s, there has been a growth of a more virulent strain this century across the growing European Union. Throughout Europe, there have been increasing concerns about the spread of infections and a noticeable variance in preventative measures.

As a result, the European Commission Directorate General for Health and Consumer Protection has funded a major project, Improving Patient Safety in Europe (IPSE; 2007), to resolve any differences through promoting standards for practice and education. The standards for practice were released in May 2007 (IPSE 2007) and cover all healthcare settings, which in the future will include hospitals, intermediate care centres, care homes, healthcare centres and polyclinics. In the near future, IPSE intends to release findings of other projects such as a feasibility study of surveillance of healthcare-acquired infections in European nursing homes, and a core

---

Box 7.1 Internet links to departments for health and social care in the devolved UK countries

- England: http://www.dh.gov.uk
- Scotland: http://www.scotland.gov.uk/health
- Wales: http://new.wales.gov.uk/topics/health/?lang=en
- Northern Ireland: http://www.dhsspsni.gov.uk/hss

curriculum for infection control practitioners (IPSE 2007). These important milestones reflect the need for more surveillance as European countries move from a hospital-centred delivery of healthcare for LTCs to one of a community setting, which will be the future. The infection control standards will enhance the national minimum standards originally published under Section 23(1) of the Care Standards Act 2000, especially Standards 19–26: the environment (Department of Health [DH] 2003). It is important to note that the introduction of devolved governments has affected the way and pace with which recommendations have been introduced. Box 7.1 provides the web links for more information on the departments of health plans for health and social care in the individual UK countries.

For many years, there has been a need to consider cost-effective ways of delivering an NHS for a nation that is living longer and placing more demands on the service. At the beginning of this century, the interim report of Wanless (2001) called for a more cost-effective way of providing a health service by 'providing services based on scientific knowledge to all who could benefit and refraining from providing services to those not likely to benefit' (p. 42). Such a statement gives power to medical knowledge but little credence to evolving social and person-centred knowledge, or to how the advance of IT could transform the service in the future. Decisions based on science alone will not work as the changing world is becoming complex and other indicators need to be included.

This report came at a time when the *National Service Framework for Older People* (DH 2001) was released. Standard 2 of this National Service Framework (NSF) raised the importance of person-centred care and the service user's voice in determining the commissioning, provision and organisation of health and social care in the future. This is increasingly seen as a more democratic approach in which individual service users are more active rather than passive in decision-making processes (Andrews et al. 2004). The NSF also raised the need for a Single Assessment Process (SAP), which is an holistic assessment tool focused on an individual's health and welfare needs. The SAP has since been adopted as a generic model for the Common Assessment Framework, which is aimed at serving all adults and not just the older person (DH 2006a). It is this framework, built with user participation, that offers a rounded assessment of both the health and social care needs of the patient. Specific information from the SAP may need to be shared with many agencies in order to support the older person in the community. The challenge for the SAP remains for those individuals living within country borders where the delivery for health is in one country and the social care is in another one. This tests the communication systems in place, but could identify the need for further systems that communicate across boundaries.

With the new NHS plans comes the need for more partnership working between many new agencies such as the Department for Communities and Local Government. Its Supporting People programme commenced in 2003 with public participation in identifying need 'to improve the delivery of housing related support to service users' (Department for Communities and Local Government 2007: 4). This new agency is still evolving, but its mission is to work in partnership with 'local authorities, service providers and service users' (p. 7), to meet the housing needs of the most vulnerable members of society. The service providers also include primary care trusts (PCTs) who will need systems in place to collate need identified by the SAP. The inclusion of health in such partnerships is important if older people with LTCs are to be enabled, with appropriate support, to remain independent in the community (Godfrey et al. 2004). Garwood (2005) has suggested that the partnership between health, housing and initiatives such as telecare and the utilisation of SAPs requires further research to monitor the effectiveness and issues evolving, otherwise there could a 'dilution of success in achieving the objectives of SAP – to the detriment of older people' (p. 20). The main detriment would be the loss of integrated, seamless care.

The SAP was also to be an important tool for the advanced primary nurses involved in the testing of case management models, which paved the way for the new community matron role (Hudson and Moore 2006). The role was to case-manage older patients with complex LTCs. One of the initiatives tested was based on the American Evercare model. As can be seen by the principles in Box 7.2, it is an holistic model that could be served by IT systems to be planned in the Connecting for Health IT programme (see below and Useful websites at the end of the chapter). The advanced primary nurse projects were introduced with little consideration for the educational needs of the nurses (Hudson and Moore 2006). Although there were tangible outcomes reported which reflected most of the principles, it is fair to say that valuable lessons were learnt from the projects and the participants' evaluations, which have informed and updated professional Advanced Practice Awards (Hudson and Moore 2006).

In considering how the principles identified in Standard 2 of the NSF (DH 2001) have embedded, it is important to explore whether or not older people are being empowered.

> **Box 7.2 The five fundamental principles of the Evercare model (reproduced with permission from Hudson and Moore, 2006)**
>
> 1. Application of an individualised, whole person approach to maximise function, independence and quality of life
> 2. Primary care will be central rather than peripheral
> 3. Keep older people out of hospital by utilising a proactive rather than reactive approach to managing health care, assisted by specific tools and techniques
> 4. Medications management and review
> 5. Robust approach to identifying, proactively managing, and monitoring the outcomes of the high-risk caseload

The empowerment of patients through the Expert Patients Programme

As discussed in Chapter 3, there is an expected shift towards the autonomy paradigm for healthcare in which expert patients will gain a 'greater moral authority' (Youngson 2008: 6) and have the confidence to work in partnership with their GPs. However, this requires a relationship of 'shared decision making and responsibility' (Coulter 1999: 719).

At least 2 years before the publication of the NSF (DH 2001), Coulter (1999) reported that paternalism in the NHS was 'endemic' owing to a culture of patient passiveness and medical control. In a bid to help people with LTCs improve their quality of life, the government planned to support an Expert Patients Programme (DH 1999, 2006b). The programme originated from the research of Lorig et al. (1993) at Stanford University, USA. Their work focused on people with arthritis, and the programme's philosophy was based on Bandura's social cognitive theory of behaviour. According to Bandura (1977), an important step towards behaviour change was the improvement of self-efficacy, the gaining of confidence and a positive attitude through taking actions. The Stanford course was lay-led as this was seen to be a cheaper option than employing healthcare professionals (Lorig et al. 1993). The programme was seen as a toolkit that enabled participants to explore self and consider alternative ways of coping with their condition, including problem-solving, ways of communicating and working with healthcare professionals, and action planning.

Following success in the USA, Donaldson (2001) felt that the UK NHS and patients would benefit from a similar programme. Prior to the implementation of the centrally controlled programme in 2002 in the UK, there had been specialist health education programmes run by professionals and not lay people. Wilson et al. (2006a) concluded in their research that although the UK programme reinforced the biomedical paradigm, there was the possibility that it was 'triggering a health consumer movement, which as a lay-initiative gives further voice to the patient narrative' (p. 30).

This may raise concerns for those professionals not willing to let go of traditional power, who do not want the patient to ask questions or who are naive regarding the effects of shifting paradigms. Wilson et al. (2006b) also reported that, of the many professionals participating in focus groups, it was the nurses who appeared more anxious about expert patients, who expressed unfounded fears of litigation and who were limited in the skills of facilitating self-management. These results may reflect a need for further education and training, but may also reflect the existence of the paternalism referred to by Coulter (1999). The gap in the education needs for health professionals and carers was also identified by the national group pioneering the Expert Patients Programme. In 2007, the Self Care for Primary Care programme was released (see Useful websites at the end of the chapter). This is aimed at PCT and social care organisations, GP and pharmacy teams. The previously known Expert Carers' Programme was redesigned and launched in August 2008 as the Caring with Confidence Programme (Carers UK 2008).

Some scepticism from medical professionals of the value of rolling out a lay-led Expert Patients Programme before robust formal evaluations have been completed is cited in the literature, the main concerns being that there is no proof of the impact of the programme on the disease process or quality of life (Buszewicz et al. 2006; Griffiths et al. 2007). However, the authors do agree that there is ample evidence of the positive impact on the patients' self-efficacy, although Griffiths et al. (2007) state that a main disappointment is that the 'use of health care has remained stubbornly unaltered' (p. 1255). Suggestions for this include that, with improved communication skills with practitioners, the patients may consult more; the current programmes do not include any correction of 'erroneous health beliefs' or 'specific disease management skills' (p. 1256). Such suggestions may need to be weighed against the fact that, according to Bandura (1977), self-efficacy is an early stage in behaviour change, and therefore more time needs to be considered for the embedding process. Even with more time, it may not be easy to determine whether the programme in isolation is effective or whether it is a contributing and supporting mechanism of many, as patients may be accessing more aids in the future such as telecare and IT information.

According to the DH (2006b) report, the Expert Patients Programme was to be increased, and the responsibility for the marketing and delivery would be removed from central government control to the new Expert

Patients Programme Community Interest Company (see Useful websites at the end of the chapter). This is a social enterprise organisation that will be responsible for developing new partnerships with PCTs and other agencies to develop new courses to meet the needs of all stakeholders (DH 2006a). The future here could be more online access for individual courses where some patients may not be able to access face-to-face group work. These of course could be exclusive for the older people who have yet to engage with IT, but it could serve as another choice to support diversity of needs. Choice regarding the delivery of future programmes must remain, as the face-to-face support of group work may be more beneficial to older people. The challenge for the future could be the development of partnership working between the Expert Patients Programme Community Interest Company and PCTs to commission the programme according to need, and not be negatively influenced by professional paternalism and control.

Community hospitals

Outlined in *Delivering Care Closer to Home* (DH 2008a) is the strategic vision to provide more services in local communities closer to people's homes, and to provide more choice and give people a say in how their local health service is shaped through Local Involvement Networks (LINks) (DH 2008b), formerly Patient and Public Involvement forums and the Commission for Patient and Public Involvement in Health. Community hospitals are ideal 'one-stop' shops for the older person to access healthcare locally without having to travel distances to a local district general hospital. Sadly in England, many community hospitals are under threat of closure, which is at odds with the government's push to bring and keep services in the community. The reasons for this are numerous, but for many PCTs the greatest costs are staffing costs, the need to make many community hospitals 'disability compliant' and the difficulty of keeping old buildings clean and free from infection with walls and ceilings that are 'dust collectors'. Many community hospitals were old manor houses, or workhouses built in the 19th century and clearly not designed with 21st-century healthcare in mind. Many are listed buildings, which would cost thousands of pounds to upgrade to ensure access for all. In many instances, the cost of refurbishment is too high and the PCTs are left with the only option open to them: closure.

In some areas, the closure of community hospitals has been the catalyst for community action. In Gloucestershire, the community successfully managed to reverse the closure of the Dilke Hospital in Cinderford. The hospital serves a rural community in the northern area of the Forest of Dean (which in total covers 110 square kilometres), and its closure would have led to just one community hospital serving the needs of the community of approximately 80,000 people. It was also proposed to hand over the remaining community hospital at Lydney to a private independent consortium, leaving the population to attend one of the two district general hospitals in the county. The closure of the Dilke was expected to save upwards of £1 million, a not insignificant sum. Through protests, demonstrations and community action, the Dilke was saved and is run by Forest Health Future Group, a Social Enterprise Trust.

The success of community action in the area is good news for older people as they are able to access a hospital with radiology, minor injury and specialist outpatient facilities without needing to travel to the nearest district general hospital. Older people are able to transfer to their local community hospital to continue their rehabilitation, which is helpful for family and friends, many of whom will also be older. It is comforting to be in a small community hospital where the care delivered is person centred and less stressful. However, decisions are often made by trusts and PCTs that adversely affect the local community, as the following example demonstrates.

Keynsham Hospital was a thriving community hospital half way between the cities of Bath and Bristol. The hospital had four wards, including a young disabled unit, the only one of its kind in the area. Full outpatient facilities were available, including outpatient clinics with visiting consultants, physiotherapy, radiology, nutrition and dietetics, occupational therapy and a day hospital. Its planned closure in 2006 was to prepare for the move to the new South Bristol Community Hospital, due to open in 2008. At the time of writing, the plans for this new hospital have finally been approved and building work has started. The community were promised a new 'health park' (due to open in summer 2009) on the site of the existing hospital with the transfer of several GP practices and the Keynsham clinic (a sexual health and family centre).

For the older population, the trust's decision meant that their nearest hospital was now in the cities of Bath or Bristol (8 and 7 miles away, respectively). The closure affected those older people who needed slow-stream rehabilitation as this was not now offered as an inpatient service but would continue in the community utilising community rehabilitation teams and intermediate care beds. The reality of the closure was that the community lost a vital resource, and the intermediate care and specialist community rehabilitation teams were overwhelmed and struggled to keep pace with demand (Murchland and Wake-Dyster 2006). Older people stayed longer in hospital, 'bed blocking' as there was a serious underestimation of the community services required to meet the needs. There was a need to consider the requirements of a transition service, which needed to be in place in order to effect a smooth and seamless conversion from one service to another.

Many community hospitals are being utilised as bases for community nursing, social care and rehabilitation teams. This assists with the notion of integration of both health and social care teams and makes the sharing of information easier and a reality. In Wiltshire in 2007, the amalgamation of three separate PCTs into one large PCT and the closure of several community hospitals prompted the reorganisation of community nursing into 11 neighbourhood nursing teams (Wiltshire Primary Care Trust 2007). Although the amalgamation was not without its problems, the positive aspects included a Single Point of Access (SPA) to bring all the multiple access points such as Rapid Response and community rehabilitation (to name but two) together. SPA is available 24 hours a day, 7 days a week, is based at a local community hospital and is reached by a single telephone number, e-referral and fax. Referrals are for both inpatient admission and community health and social care teams. This is a prime example of how bringing services closer to the community can be of benefit for the older person, although change is not easy to deal with whether you are 45 or 85 years old. Not having to contact different providers and make numerous telephone calls is very helpful for an older person who may be muddled or confused by all the different individuals he or she may need to contact. It should also avoid duplication and wasted resources.

Other ways to bring services to the community are by mobile screening and treatment units. Mobile breast screening units, retinopathy screening units, podiatry services and mobile X-ray units are now a familiar sight in many communities and able to take services out to isolated areas. Older people will greatly benefit from these units, particularly the retinopathy and podiatry services. Older people are at risk from missing health checks and screening appointments, particularly if they are housebound and isolated. The continuation of these services is vital for older people to maintain and improve their quality of life.

Cancer care – bringing diagnostic technology and chemotherapy treatment closer to patients

In the past, older people living in rural areas have often faced long journeys of approximately 60–70 miles to visit hospitals for either diagnostic technology such as positron emission tomography (PET scanning) or chemotherapy treatment. Although the journey alone can be tiring, the interventions can also have a negative impact for those with lung cancer and diabetes.

In preparation for the PET scan, patients are starved for 6 hours and on arrival spend at least 2 hours with the radiographer during the procedure before returning home. The procedure includes the injection of a radioactive, sugary compound called 18-fluorodeoxyglucose. The patient is expected to drink four or five glasses of water, which helps to flush the tracer, and to rest prior to the scan. Within the hospital environment, there are the amenities and space to deal with an older person who may have a leaking wound or problems with continence, breathing or claustrophobia. However, these could be challenges for the teams operating the peripatetic PET/computed tomography scanners that are being introduced in parts of England, such as the Midlands. The parking of the mobile scanners has to be carefully considered for balance, access and closeness to public conveniences as they do not have toilet facilities due to the space taken up by the technology. A common site could be a community hospital, which could still mean a distance to travel for some older people.

A national cancer charity called Hope for Tomorrow (see Useful websites at the end of the chapter) was set up by a widow whose husband was stressed during his illness by the journey of 60 miles to the oncology centre in Cheltenham. In collaboration with a consultant from the Gloucestershire NHS Foundation Trust, the charity's fundraising has financed the world's first mobile chemotherapy unit. The first unit was equipped with wheelchair access, a treatment room for five patients at a time, a carer's room and the latest technology to support treatment and the comfort of patients, carers and staff. Current fundraising will fund a second vehicle to be adapted as a mobile chemotherapy assessment and support unit, which will include a blood analysis machine. These facilities will be more accessible for most patients as the siting of the vehicles will not be curtailed by the same health and safety regulations as the PET scanner. However, both of these examples of peripatetic amenities indicate how collaborative healthcare has come to meet the immediate needs of patients in the community.

Although it is a useful resource for the community, we need to be cognisant of the fact that many community hospitals are in areas that are rural or semi-rural and not always accessible without a car. This could severely disadvantage many older people, who may be reliant on public transport or family and friends to take them to the hospital.

The National Programme for IT

NHS Connecting for Health is an agency of the DH and was formed in 2005 with the prime responsibility of implementing the National Programme for IT. To guide and implement such a comprehensive and complex programme, Senior Responsible Owners were appointed for each participating region and are supported by leadership development initiatives. Further information on such initiatives can be found at the web addresses indicated in Box 7.3.

Box 7.3 Web links for support initiatives for the NHS Connecting for Health Programme

- http://www.connectingforhealth.nhs.uk/systemsandservices/capability/lisa
- http://www.espace.connectingforhealth.nhs.uk
- http://www.isip.nhs.uk
- http://www.isip.nhs.uk/bookcase
- http://www.isip.nhs.uk/case-studies/case-studies-theme

In supporting PCTs and local health community boards to take some ownership of identifying IT systems to support their capability in delivering service improvement, guidelines and the Local Health Communities Information Management and Technology Self Assessment Tool (LISA), were introduced for the Chief Executives and teams led by the Senior Responsible Owners. The strategic plan for Connecting for Health identified the northern regions to be the first to participate, with the South West Region being the last. The South West would be a bigger challenge due to the earlier failure of the Wessex Regional Information Systems Plan in 1992 (National Audit Office [NAO], 2008). This failed due to lack of commitment from trusts that is reflected by the responses of the three current local service providers, CSC, Fujitsu and BT, as one reason why there is a 4-year delay in the national project (NAO, 2008).

Other priorities of the national project were to set up electronic patient records, a choose-and-book service for outpatient appointments, a facility to transfer notes from one GP to another, an electronic prescription service, and a picture archiving and communications system. Although there have been some successes, (notably with the picture archiving systems, PACs), the NAO (2008) report has highlighted some security issues, especially concerning confidentiality, that need to be resolved before some GPs will upload patient records. Some GPs have reported that the choose-and-book system is currently too slow to be utilised in face-to-face meetings with patients, so choice is often delayed or compromised. Utilisation of the electronic resources across England ranges from 20% to 90%. There are concerns that 16% of nurses and 7% of doctors interviewed had never heard of the IT programme (NAO, 2008).

The report recognised that the programme's website (see Useful websites at the end of the chapter) celebrates the achievements to date but recommends that there needs to be more openness and realism in presenting what needs to be achieved. Awareness of the vision of a new NHS by healthcare staff and their commitment to learning from the stages of implementation of projects are priorities if the reality of efficient systems are to be in place to promote integrated care to improve standards, especially of communication between primary and secondary care.

Many older people will have used the Internet to find information about their problems and how to manage them. We need to remember that many older people are Internet-savvy. A report by Bytheway (2007) for the Research on Age Discrimination Project stated that 'there is a widespread ageist belief that older people are unable to cope with IT' (p. 1). Clearly, this is incorrect as the number of users of the Internet and technology in general is on the increase. For the 'Baby Boomers', technology such as the Internet, email and IT will be as commonplace in its usage as a telephone is today.

For the current cohort of older people, media literacy is increasing. OFCOM produced a report on media literacy among older people (those over 65 years old) in 2006. It makes interesting reading and challenges ageist assumptions that older people have no interest in IT, digital technology or mobile telephones. In the report, home use of the Internet is broadly the same for older users as for all UK adults, at 6.1 versus 6.5 hours per week. Other statistics are that:

- 68% of older people surveyed use the Internet for communication via email with family and friends
- 31% use the Internet for work or study information
- 32% use it for transactions such as Internet banking and shopping
- 27% use it for news
- 28% use the Internet for entertainment and leisure activities such as editing photographs and quizzes.

With the exception of work and study and entertainment, these figures are comparable to those of the UK adult population overall. Computer literacy is rated highly among older users. It would seem perfectly reasonable then to assume that many older people will be more than capable of searching the Internet for health information, will be able to book appointments online and, in the move towards telecare and telehealth, be easily able to cope with the technology required to send information either via a computer or a telephone line.

Telecare, telehealth, telenursing and telemedicine

IT is not new to community care as the NHS Direct initiative was introduced in 1998. The introduction was prompted by a need for gate-keeping for primary care services and to reduce inappropriate attendance at Accident and Emergency departments. It is a 24-hour service that offers advice and generally directs the caller to their nearest most appropriate primary care service. In situations where GPs do not have an 'out of hours' triage system in place, it also covers this facility. This is a form of telephone triage where nurses from a distance assess patients' needs during the out of hours period when their GPs are not available, but a small service is provided in a nearby town or city. It was introduced to reduce the costs of inappropriate face-to-face consultation. To enable the nurses based in call centres to make accurate assessments and to give advice or refer the patient to the out of hours GP, computer programmes based on medical algorithms were developed. These formed a series of problem-solving questions, the answers to which should enable the nurse to build a picture of the patient and his or her pathology and environment (Edwards 1998).

According to Snooks et al. (2008) the introduction of this form of telenursing has caused 'conflicts' (p. 637) and maybe 'rifts' (p. 638) between community nurses giving face-to-face care and those working at a distance through NHS Direct. The main concerns identified by Snooks et al. were that community nurses and some NHS Direct nurses questioned whether this was 'real' nursing and whether the communication skills of nurses working in isolation were highly developed. Such concerns regarding the IT alternative to nurse–patient consultations were also expressed by Pascoe and Neal (2004). Snooks et al. recommended that if telenursing were to contribute to the vision of integrated care, any gaps in the perception of the role needed to be addressed by further research. They also suggested a need for the introduction of 'split roles' (p. 639), between the face-to-face and distant approaches in order to provide a better understanding of the value of both situations in providing integrated care. This suggestion may arise from the need for more time and evidence during a time of embedding new processes. Experienced nurses may give a different response to the role of nurses working in call centres such as NHS Direct.

Findings from a recent research project by McGill (2008), who interviewed part-time but experienced nurses working in an independent call centre serving a group of GP practices, suggest that with experience the telenursing approach may be filling gaps occurring during paradigm shifts of healthcare. Generally, clinical symptoms were assessed accurately on the computerised system, but the nurses were critical of the IT package, which was based on medical language and decision trees alone, and whose outcomes could be misleading if nurses kept rigidly to the tree of questions.

There may be other influences that professionals may need to consider when using such packages. Groopman (2007: 5) identified that 'algorithms discourage physicians from thinking independently and creatively'. So this could constrain a doctor from thinking outside the disease box to consider where the patient was 'coming from'. To think creatively, a professional will need to pull eclectic information together in order to paint the patient's picture. Without this, there is a possibility of misdiagnosis.

An example identified by McGill (2008) was the word 'confusion', which was first identified by the algorithm as a mental health problem. Instead, by further holistic questioning, the nurse suspected an underlying urinary tract infection. Overall, the nurses found that by, altering their language and communication and assessment skills, they identified many social circumstances and differing levels of support in the home environment, which affected their decision-making to bring the patient in for a face-to-face consultation – or not. They identified that 'at-risk' groups such as the older person and those requiring palliative care might be socially isolated and their medical needs complex. Therefore, they were more likely to need face-to-face assessment as it was difficult to make decisions regarding risk management and ascertain the severity of the patients' symptoms over the telephone. Further gaps in the system were identified within palliative care in the community, where worried relatives contacted the call centre concerned about lack of pain control and issues of comfort. This was quite distressing where night-sitters and professional night cover had not been available, especially in rural areas (McGill 2008).

Communication gaps between professionals, patients and informal carers are well documented, and IT does offer a possible means of synergy, although this will only happen when professionals use the SAP effectively and start to work in partnership with other agencies. This is already happening in some parts of the UK.

Next we explore examples of where some GPs are working with other agencies to use technology to help prevent hospitalisation and aid vital signs monitoring. Local authorities are being aided by government grants to use the new technologies to manage risks and redeploy care where the need is greatest at certain times of the year.

Scenario 7.1: New technology

A 72-year-old man lives alone in a bungalow and is practically house-bound owing to COPD. He is a very independent man and receives help for shopping and house care from social services; he also relies on Meals-on-Wheels. His neighbour helps him with his medications and collects his prescriptions from the local pharmacy. During the next winter months, his neighbour plans to take a cruise so the community matron is contacted to review the patient's support mechanisms. It is during these months that the patient often experiences exacerbation of his condition and has in the past required hospitalisation.

The Eurowinter Group led by Keatinge and Donaldson (1997) undertook many surveys across Europe between 1988 to 1994 to establish whether 'increases in mortality per 1°C fall in temperature differ in various European regions and to relate any differences to usual winter climate and measures to protect against cold' (p. 1341). Even though it was known that cold stress had a negative effect on individual patients' immunity and resilience to winter ailments, the surveys showed that often older people did not wear sufficient layers to keep warm and were not particularly active out of doors. It was this research that inspired the Meteorological Office to work collaboratively with a Finnish telemedicine company to pioneer COPD health forecasting in 2004 (Bewley 2008). This is a fully automated service that makes calls five times a year when adverse weather is forecast. The main automated questions are:

• Do you have enough medication for your COPD to last for the next 2 weeks?
• Have your symptoms become worse than normal?

The patients' responses are logged onto the system, which alerts GP practices via email to log on and view the results. If the patients do not answer the telephone calls, a further three attempts are made to make contact with them. This information is also logged on to the system. Any follow-ups are made at the discretion of the practice. Some, for example, deploy a community matron or district nurse, or prescribe further medication for a local pharmacist to deliver.

The pilot for the work in the UK was in the winter of 2006/07 in Cornwall and was financed by the Cornwall Adult Social Care and Cornwall PCT. A total of 447 patients with COPD were recruited to the programme and consented to their details being entered onto the NHS Net. Each patient was provided with a guide to health forecasting that had some seasonal advice to avoid infections, colds and overheating, and some useful telephone and web links. The evaluation consisted of 345 completed questionnaires, with 89% of respondents stating that the calls were helpful and 11% not helpful. The actions taken in response to the calls included:

• 30% of respondents consulting the patient information pack provided
• 19% consulting their GP
• 53% obtaining a repeat prescription.

A further evaluation of hospital admissions showed rates of 54% lower in the practices involved in the project, and they were down by 52% when compared with the previous year. It was forecast that if the programme was rolled out across Cornwall, the reduction in admissions could generate up to £300,000 in savings (Bewley 2008). Following this pilot, the system has been contracted by eight PCTs across England, Wales and Scotland.

This multiagency case study is but one of many that are evolving as scientists and private companies are working closer with healthcare professionals to devise ways of supporting and monitoring vulnerable older people in the community. As local health needs assessments become more efficient, it is possible to see a growth in such technologies that will help managers to deploy staff effectively according to the health needs of the patients, especially in rural communities such as Cornwall.

Building telecare in England (DH 2005)

In July 2004, the government announced plans to invest £80 million over 2 years from April 2006 through the Preventative Technology Grant. The purpose of the grant was to initiate a change in the design and delivery of health, social care and housing services by using telecare as a prevention strategy to enhance and maintain the well-being and independence of individuals. This is an ideal solution for the older person in order for them to stay in their home in situations that would in the past have meant admission to hospital or a nursing home

Telecare

There appears to be no real consensus on what telecare is, but 'telecare' describes any service that brings health and social care directly to users, usually in their own homes, and which is supported by information and communication technology (ICT) in order to manage the risks associated with independent living (NHS Institute for Innovation and Improvement and Kent County Council 2006). It is sometimes referred to as 'assistive technology'. Telehealth is a component of telecare. Telecare Aware (see Useful websites at the end of the chapter) list a number of examples of Telecare devices (Box 7.4).

Telemedicine

The following definition, by the World Health Organization (2008: 1), states that:

Telemedicine is the use of telecommunication technologies to provide healthcare services across geographic, ... social, and cultural barriers. It is the delivery of healthcare services, [remotely] by healthcare professionals using information and communications technologies for the exchange of valid information for diagnosis, treatment and prevention of diseases and injuries, research and evaluation, and for the continuing education of healthcare providers, all in the interest of advancing health and their communities.

Box 7.4 Types of telecare device

Movement/non-movement sensors
Fire/smoke alarms
Food/water alarms
Window/door sensors
Bed/chair occupancy sensors
Gas shut-off devices
Wrist-worn well-being monitors and
personal pendant alarms

Falls sensors
Automatic lighting sensors
Fridge activity sensors
Carbon monoxide sensors
Temperature range sensors
Medication reminder systems
Safety confirmation devices

Telehealth

Telehealth monitoring is the remote exchange of physiological data between a patient at home and medical or nursing staff in the hospital or GP surgery, to assist in diagnosis and monitoring. It could include a home unit to measure and monitor temperature, blood pressure, blood glucose, cardiac arrhythmias or lung function for clinical review at a remote location (for example, a hospital site) using telephone lines or wireless technology.

e-Health

e-Health refers to the use of ICT to meet needs of citizens, patients, healthcare professionals and healthcare providers, by providing health-related activities, services and systems carried out over a distance for the purposes of health promotion, disease education, management and research for health. Via this e-health system the individual will be able to interact with the healthcare provider, receive education and be empowered to take greater control of his or her own health and healthcare.

Box 7.5 Examples of use of ICT for e-healthcare

Remote monitoring of health and biological signs	Self-help programmes, e.g. Dry Out Now (see Chapter 4)	Remotely monitored preventative help
Health assessment online	Electronic patient records	Remote consultation
Online health forums, blogs and wikis	Direct communication with healthcare professionals	Health education and health enquiry services

---

The Telemedicine Alliance was formed under the auspices of the European Commission within the Information Society Technologies Directorate. The overall goal was to formulate an underlying policy for the application of e-health in support of the European citizen, and to create a 'vision' for a personal healthcare network by the year 2010. Some examples of e-healthcare are provided in Box 7.5.

For more information about telecare, telehealth and telemedicine, access the Care Services Improvement Partnership web pages (listed at the end of the chapter), which have some good up-to-date information, fact sheets and newsletters.

There is still some way to go before seamless care is perfected. The following examples are of differing strategies to work towards seamless care.

Whole System Demonstrators

Whole System Demonstrators in Kent, Cornwall and Newham, London, were selected by the DH to take forward integration of health and social care supported by advanced assistive technology (telehealth and telecare; see Useful websites at the end of the chapter).

Kent has probably been one of the most successful of the demonstrators, which has been helped by a dynamic and forward-thinking council director. Kent's increasing ageing population and diminishing workforce were the impetus for the Whole System Demonstrators. The use of technology such as telehealth and telecare were seen as one of the ways of supporting older people to remain in their own homes. In Kent, typical telehealth monitoring equipment includes a blood pressure, a blood glucose and a pulse oximetry monitor. Each patient has an electronic hub where they upload readings daily and send them to a clinical team via a secure web link. This is read by the nurse, and the patient is contacted and given advice. The messages are sent electronically through the hub or via video telephone, or ordinary telephone conversations with the community nursing teams.

The advantages for the older person are that the feedback is responsive and quick. They are reassured and empowered to self-manage. Individuals have greater understanding of their disease and their health. Careful and close daily monitoring means that subtle changes in the individuals' condition are picked up very quickly and acted upon before the change leads to a more serious event. Kent provides a nice example of this: 'We have one lady, for instance who tends to add as little as a kilo just two or three days before having a cardiac arrhythmia. If the care team had only weekly data to go on the chances are they'd miss this and she would run into problems' (NHS Institute for Innovation and Improvement and Kent County Council 2006: 5).

We need to be cognisant of the fact that, for many people, telecare or the use of assistive technology may be perceived as unethical. Thorough and person-centred assessment will ascertain exactly what assistive technology might be useful. Chapter 6 highlighted some examples of this. The COPD scenario above is a very good example of where the technology has assisted the older person to remain independent and is not perceived in a negative way.

Integration of health and social services is the next stage that will assist the move towards seamless care. Here we provide two examples of where integrated and seamless care have been facilitated and championed and are working effectively. In visiting both of these examples, we saw at first hand how a dynamic leader with vision helps to move ideas and solutions forward.

Moving towards seamless care

West Lothian Community Health and Care Partnership (CHCP) Scotland

West Lothian set up a partnership between community health, social services and housing (the council). In common with other health and social care providers in the four countries of the UK, there was a need for 'radical change in policies for the care and support of older people . . . focused on care at home . . . a radical rethink of services' (Bowes and McColgan 2006). West Lothian wanted to provide a more equitable and effective service with a view to having a 'one-stop shop approach' that would be managed by one director. West Lothian aimed to reduce the number of unplanned medical admissions, minimise length of stay and support early discharge back into the community for older people aged 65 years or more with two or more unplanned admissions in the previous year. The use of technology and an integrated approach to care was considered vital to move these ideas forward.

West Lothian (2001 census) has:

- 25,800 people aged 60 and over = 16.2% of the West Lothian population
- a 2004–24 projected rate of increase = 72% compared with 39% in Scotland as a whole.

A project manager was responsible for setting up the Strathbrock Partnership Centre and bringing together in one centre a series of managers responsible for discharge, re-enablement and technology.

Strathbrock Partnership Centre West Lothian

Strathbrock Partnership Centre in West Lothian opened in 2002, serves a population of approximately 35,000, and is a purpose-built building with 12 partners occupying the block. The first impressions of the centre are that it is airy, clean, vast and well used by the community. The centre houses:

- a pharmacy, which offers a delivery service as well as on-site dispensing
- the Café Mistura, operated by Capability Scotland, which is open to staff and members of the public
- housing services – rent and council tax can be paid here, and requests for housing repairs made
- a council information service
- a health centre of three GP practices and community nursing teams, health visitors and midwives
- a justice centre
- physiotherapy, occupational therapy and technology, speech and language therapy, and podiatry services
- the base for the community equipment manager
- a re-enablement team
- mental health nursing teams and a mental health resource centre
- a social work department
- Carers of West Lothian, providing support, information and guidance
- community adult education in conjunction with West Lothian College
- a community centre, which includes a playgroup, children's clubs and dance classes.

The advantages of the system

The partnership centre uses a shared information system, thus enabling the smooth transfer of information between different providers (as outlined in the SAP). The older person will not need to share information with several different people as the information is recorded, stored and shared (with permission) between the different providers.

The single point of access is helpful for the community as a whole, particularly for older people. The older person will not need to visit several different buildings and departments in order to resolve problems. There is also an information desk with a range of information available. Appointments can be made here to save the older person having to queue more than once.

Having all services in one building means that, in a typical visit, the older person could discuss housing issues with a housing officer, see the GP or practice nurse, collect a prescription from the pharmacy, see a social worker and have a snack and drink in the welcoming café without needing to move out of the building. A bus service serves the centre, and proposed plans include adding other services such as community police officers and, it is hoped, a cash machine.

For the staff, working together in one building advances the ethos of integrated and shared working. All services are together and information can be shared quickly and easily through the shared information system and through joined-up thinking and working. Referrals are made directly to the relevant service and, within 48 hours of being informed of a discharge, an older person could be at home with a full safety package and other equipment. This is impressive and should be the standard that all integrated teams work towards. Staff appear to get on well together and are enabled and empowered to make decisions without needing innumerable referrals to different teams, different managers and multiple assessments. There are still problems with secondary and acute care not sharing information quickly enough with the community teams, which will delay discharges, but there is no doubt that this will be resolved in the near future.

Telecare

West Lothian CHCP is a prolific user of telecare, which it utilises in over 3500 homes and supported housing environments. The purpose of the technology, as stated on their website, is to 'provide an innovative form of housing for older people with support needs that will sustain independent living through effective physical design, focused individual care planning and the efficient use of new technologies'. There are three levels of technology, described below.

The *Home Safety Service* is the largest group, with a 'core package of technology' fitted in individuals' own homes:

- The home alarm unit provides two-way speech, and all other sensors are radio-triggered to the unit. It sends calls to a call centre staffed 24 hours a day with trained telecare operators who action the calls
- Smoke detector alarms within the home send an alarm to the call centre
- Extreme temperature sensors pick up both high and low temperatures
- Two flood detectors are included – one for the bathroom and one in the kitchen – the technology being such that the call centre can tell which of the two has been triggered, which means a faster response to correct the problem
- The activity detectors are passive infrared sensors and are used both to monitor activity and as a home security system.

The cost is around (at the time of publication) £300 and is met by the CHCP.

Home Safety Service Plus is a second-level package with the basic Home Safety equipment as well as additional equipment that is individual to the customer's needs, for example devices to detect wandering, video door entry systems, chair or bed occupancy monitors, carbon monoxide detectors and voice recognition systems.

Housing with Care is a third-level package and used by tenants supported in the Housing with Care tenancies, who have a core package of the Home Safety technology, a personal pendant alarm, a video door entry system and pull emergency cords. Other technology is offered based on individual assessments but could include, for example, an activity reminder such as pill times uploaded onto the telephone, which will ring at an allotted time. When the older person answers, they will hear a familiar voice such as a family member reminding them to take the medication, go back to bed, etc.. The cost of providing the technology in the Housing with Care tenancies is included in the weekly rent.

Advantages of telecare

For the older person, the advantages are enormous. People with multiple and complex needs can be managed successfully at home with the use of technology such as that described above. Older people may take some time to get used to the technology, but it is clear that if used effectively and tailored to the older person's needs, the potential benefit is enormous.

For community staff, there is a real shift of thinking. The older person is empowered to remain independent at home, and staff therefore need to question their former ways of working, to focus on promoting independence for older people and to provide 'support' rather than 'care'.

Professional boundaries are blurred, and there is more sharing of tasks formerly separated (Bailey 2004). The growth and advances in technology mean that community nurses will have to radically rethink their working practices in order to use their skills and time more effectively. Remote monitoring will mean that more advanced skills, including the application of diagnostic criteria and the interpretation of physiological parameters, will need to be developed.

Torbay Care Trust

The Care Trust was formed in December 2005 after the integration of Torbay PCT and adult social services, formerly provided by Torbay Council, a unitary authority. The trust provides community healthcare services including Brixham and Paignton Community Hospitals, adult social care and learning disability services. The trust is divided into five areas: Brixham, Paignton North and South, and Torquay North and South.

Paignton Community Hospital houses an inpatient unit, a minor injuries unit and radiology and physiotherapy services, and is the base for Paignton North and South integrated health and social care teams. Brixham Community Hospital has a minor injuries unit, two inpatient wards, occupational therapy, outpatient facilities, physiotherapy, podiatry, speech and language therapy and X-ray services, and is the base for Brixham integrated health and social care teams.

Each zone serves a population of approximately 23,000 people (with the exception of Torquay South, which serves a population of 45,000). This doubles in the summer months to include the transient tourist population. Each zone has a general manager who is supported by a professional lead for each of the disciplines, i.e. nursing, physiotherapy, occupational therapy and social work. Each zone has a community matron. Within each discipline are teams that deliver the care assisted by support workers trained to NVQ level 3 or 4. Each zone team covers all services – intermediate care, palliative care and Rapid Response and community nursing. Therapy staff move between the community hospital and the community, ensuring that needs are responded to and staff are used appropriately.

Advantages of the system

Like West Lothian, Torbay has a single point of contact and access. Prior to this set-up, the service was fragmented and confusing, and the older person or care professional may have needed to telephone several different numbers to get the requisite service. This resulted in a duplication of services and, in the worst case scenario, no service at all as there was little coordination of information between services and little ownership of problems.

The single point of access is staffed by a health and social care coordinator (not a registered practitioner) who triages telephone calls and coordinates services, ensuring the individual is referred to the most appropriate professional. Social care, social workers, therapy and nursing staff in each zone are all based centrally. Home care coordinators are also on hand to quickly set up care packages. The service is needs led and efficient. Resources are pooled and shared. Response times are quick, and patients are seen the same day. Equipment can be delivered the same day to enable an older person to get home quickly.

Staff are motivated, and there is investment in training and education. Support workers complete a comprehensive package of training across the health and social care spectrum including mental health needs and medication assistance (such as administration of insulin). Staff numbers are high with large numbers of therapy and social work staff to cover each zone.

The future

Investment in staff development of advanced skills for registered and qualified staff is key to the success of these integrated teams. Changes in working practices have not always been easy or smooth. There was and still is resistance from some GPs, social workers and community nurses. There are some areas of development such as shared care folders that have not worked as effectively as hoped as staff have not completed the information. Access to patient notes and information has been patchy in some areas of the trust. Some GP surgeries have been reluctant to share this information across the teams. The nursing service is going through a period of transition with changing shift patterns in response to the changing needs of the community. There are still problems to overcome with discharge from secondary care, which is leaving referrals too late. Despite these issues it is clear that Torbay Care trust have integrated teams that work effectively for the benefit of the community, and positively for the older person. In December 2008 the trust won a prestigious national award for the quality of service it provides for patients requiring long term care, recognition for the difference the teams have made to the older person and to others with a long term condition.

Partnership for Older People Projects

The ethos of the Partnership for Older People Projects (POPP; Care Services Improvement Partnership 2006) is to focus on promoting independence in older people by giving them choice and control, in order to enable them to avoid emergency hospital visits and to live longer independently. The £60 million grant encourages councils in England in partnership with the local NHS trust, PCT and voluntary and community sector to develop innovative approaches to supporting older people in active and healthy living. The POPP programme comprises 29 pilot sites. The first round of 19 sites started in May 2006 and the second round of a further 10 sites commenced in May 2007. The sites are varied in their approaches, but there is an emphasis on:

- providing more low-level care and support in the community to prevent or delay the need for more intense and costly care
- reducing avoidable emergency admissions to hospital
- supporting more older people to live at home or in supported housing rather than in long-term residential care
- provide person-centred and integrated care for older people
- approaches that promote health, well-being and independence for older people.

There are key areas that cut across all POPP projects. These are:

- rights
- choice
- information
- empowerment.

Examples of POPP projects

More details of the POPP projects can be found on the POPP website (see Useful websites at the end of the chapter), but two examples are outlined below.

North Somerset: integrated community health and social care services

This project will include Single Point of Access and share assessment processes and information systems. The integrated teams will include mental health, community nursing and adult social care services clustered into four teams. What is unique to this project, however, is the post of community development worker for older people, who will be employed and managed by Age Concern. Their role will be to target the isolated older person, encourage participation in volunteer schemes and befriending services, and encourage self-help.

Devon: My Life, My Choice – Feeling Good at Home in Devon

The project contains three elements:

- multidisciplinary teams
- community mentors
- foot care services,

The project will see the development of a multidisciplinary care pathway across services provided by primary, social, voluntary sector and community care. As we have seen previously, this is another form of integrated care and is likely to be a positive change for older people. The community mentors will work with older people who have become isolated or lost confidence, hard to reach groups, minority ethnic elders and carers. The mentors will encourage independence and participation in the community either as individuals or as part of a group. The foot care service will support volunteers to carry out a toenail cutting service and provide a fast track referral to a podiatrist.

Conclusion

In *Delivering Care Closer to Home* (DH 2008a: 2), three challenges are outlined:

- Bringing care closer to home in a way that both involves people as partners in designing services and delivering their care, and which reaches all of the population, addressing inequalities;
- Ensuring that services closer to home form part of integrated care pathways for users, making effective links between health, social care and other services;
- Building commissioning capacity and capability, working with communities to establish the outcomes that matter to them and the most appropriate ways of meeting them.

These three areas will shape the community health and social care practice of the future. The community nurses of the future may well visit more people virtually rather than actually in their own homes. They will be working with and empowering older people using technology not just to monitor changes in health, but also to diagnose, support, manage health conditions and send information remotely to a specialist centre. There will be concerns about losing the 'human touch' (Tweddle 2008) but these are unfounded. Interpersonal skills will need to be used in different ways without always the benefit of face-to-face contact. Community nurses will need to embrace these changes and are in a unique position to take this forward.

References

Andrews, J.A., Manthorpe, J. and Watson, R. (2004) Involving older people in intermediate care. *Journal of Advanced Nursing* 46(3): 303–10.

Bailey, S. (2004) Nursing knowledge in integrated care. *Nursing Standard* 18(44): 38–41.

Bandura, A. (1977) Self efficacy: toward a unifying theory of behavioural change. *Psychology Review* 84(2): 191–215.

Bewley, N. (2008) *Reducing Hospital Admissions Using Health Forecasting.* Conference Paper presented at the CHAIN Telehealth Networking Event, Warwick University.

Bowes, A. and McColgan, G. (2006) *Smart Technology and Community Care for Older People: Innovation in West Lothian, Scotland.* Edinburgh: Age Concern.

Buszewicz, M., Rait, G., Griffin, M. et al. (2006) Self management of arthritis in primary care: randomised controlled trial. *British Medical Journal* 333(7574): 879–85.

Bytheway, B. (2007) *Older People and the Internet. A report from the Research on Age Discrimination Project (RoAD).* Available from http://www.open.ac.uk/hsc/research/research-projects/road/the-road-reports.php.

Care Services Improvement Partnership (2006) *Partnerships for Older People Projects (POPP).* available from http://www.cat.csip.org.uk/index.cfm?pid=596.

Carers UK (2008) *Caring with Confidence.* Available from http://www.carersuk.org/Getinvolved/EqualPartners/Consultationsroundup/1218729411.

Chapman, C. (2008) This was the most dramatic period of my career. *Nursing Standard* 22(43): 19.

Coulter, A. (1999) Paternalism or partnership? *British Medical Journal* 319(7217): 719–20.

Darzi, Lord (2008) *High Quality Care for All – NHS Next Stage Review Final Report.*

Department for Communities and Local Government (2007) *Independence and Opportunity: Our Strategy for Supporting People.* Available from http://www.spkweb.org.uk/.

Department of Health (1999) *Saving Lives: Our Healthier Nation.* London: HMSO.

Department of Health (2001) *National Service Framework for Older People.* Available from http://www.dh.gov.uk/en/Publicationsandstatistics/Publications/PublicationsPolicyAndGuidance/DH_4003066.

Department of Health (2003) *Care Homes for Older People: National Minimum Standards and the Care Homes Regulations*, 3rd edn. Available from http://www.dh.gov.uk/en/Publicationsandstatistics/Publications/PublicationsPolicyAndGuidance/DH_4005819.

Department of Health (2005) *Building Telecare in England.* Available from http://www.dh.gov.uk/en/Publicationsandstatistics/Publications/PublicationsPolicyAndGuidance/DH_4115303.

Department of Health (2006a) *Our Health, Our Care, Our Say: A New Direction for Community Services.* Available from http://www.dh.gov.uk/en/Publicationsandstatistics/Publications/PublicationsPolicyAndGuidance/DH_4127453.

Department of Health (2006b) *Progress on Policy. The Expert Patients Programme*. Available from http://www.dh.gov.uk/en/Aboutus/MinistersandDepartmentLeaders/ChiefMedicalOfficer/ProgressOnPolicy/index.htm.

Department of Health (2008a) *Delivering Care Closer to Home: Meeting the Challenge*. Available from http://www.dh.gov.uk/en/Publicationsandstatistics/Publications/PublicationsPolicyandGuidance/DH_086052.

Department of Health (2008b) *Stronger Voice Better Care – Local Involvement Networks (LINks) Explained*. Available from http://www.dh.gov.uk/en/Publicationsandstatistics/Publications/PublicationsPolicyAndGuidance/DH_086056.

Donaldson, L. (2001) *The Expert Patient: A New Approach to Chronic Disease Management for the 21st Century*, HMSO: London available from http://www.dh.gov.uk/prod_consum_dh/groups/dh_digitalassets/@dh/@en/documents/digitalasset/dh_4018578.pdf.

Edwards, B. (1998) Seeing is believing – picture building: a key component of telephone triage. *Journal of Clinical Nursing* 7(1): 51–7.

Garwood, S. (2005) *Single Assessment Process and the Housing Sector – A Discussion Paper*. Available from http://www.integratedcarenetwork.gov.uk/_library/Resources/Housing/Housing_advice/Single_Assessment_Process_and_the_Housing_Sector_-_A_Discussion_Paper_-_April_2005.doc.

Godfrey, M., Townsend, J. and Denby, T. (2004) *Building a Good Life for Older People in Local Communities*. Available from http://www.jrf.org.uk/knowledge/findings/socialcare/014.asp.

Green, M. (2008) Every last thermometer was accounted for. *Nursing Standard* 22(43): 20.

Griffiths, C., Foster, G., Ramsay, J., Eldridge, S. and Taylor, S. (2007) How effective are expert patient (lay led) education programmes for chronic disease? *British Medical Journal* 334(7606): 1254.

Groopman, J. (2007) *How Doctors Think*. New York: Houghton Mifflin.

Hudson, A.J. and Moore, L.J. (2006) A new way of caring for older people in the community. *Nursing Standard* 40(26): 41–7.

Improving Patient Safety in Europe (2007) *Recommended Practices, Standards and Indicators for Monitoring the Control of HAI and AMR*. Available from http://ipse.univ-lyon1.fr.

Keatinge, W.R. and Donaldson, G.C. (1997) Cold exposure and winter mortality from ischaemic heart disease, cerebrovascular disease, respiratory disease, and all causes in warm and cold regions of Europe. *Lancet* 349(9062): 1341–6.

Lorig, K.R., Mazonson, P.D. and Holman, H.R. (1993) Evidence suggesting that health education for self-management in patients with chronic arthritis has sustained health benefits while reducing health care costs. *Arthritis and Rheumatism* 36(4): 439–46.

McGill, S. (2008) *Do Patients Exert Extraneous Influences upon Nurse's Decision Making in the Decision Support of Telephone Triage?* Unpublished MSc Dissertation, University of the West of England, Bristol.

Murchland, S. and Wake-Dyster, W. (2006) Resource allocation for community based therapy. *Disability and Rehabilitation* 28(22): 1425–32.

National Audit Office (2008) *The National Programme for IT in the NHS: Progress since 2006.* Available from http://www.official-documents.gov.uk/document/hc0708/hc04/0484/0484_i.asp.

NHS Institute for Innovation and Improvement and Kent County Council (2006) *Telehealth in Kent: What's Behind its Success?* Available from http://chain.ulcc.ac.uk/chain/documents/Telehealth_In_Kent.pdf.

OFCOM (2006) *Media Literacy Audit: Report on Media Literacy Amongst Older People.* Available from http://www.ofcom.org.uk/advice/media_literacy/medlitpub/medlitpubrss/older/.

Pascoe, S.W. and Neal, R.D. (2004) Primary care: questionnaire survey of alternative forms of patient and nurse face-to-face consultations. *Journal of Clinical Nursing* 13(3): 406–7.

Scharmer, C.O. (2007) *Theory U: Leading from the Future as it Emerges – the Social Technology of Presencing.* Cambridge, MA: Society for Organizational Learning.

Snooks, H.A., Williams, A.M., Griffiths, L.J. et al. (2008) Real nursing? The development of telenursing. *Journal of Advanced Nursing* 61(6): 631–40.

Telemedicine Alliance, *Telemedicine 2010: Visions for a Personal Medical Network.* Available from http://www.esa.int/esapub/br/br229/br229.pdf.

Tweddle, L. (2008) Will Telecare aid independence? *Nursing Times* 104(20): 8–9.

Wanless, D. (2001) *Securing our Future Health: Taking a Long Term view. Interim Report.* London: Her Majesty's Treasury.

Wilson, P.M., Kendall, S. and Brooks, F. (2006a) *The Expert Patients Programme: A Paradox of Patient Empowerment and Medical Dominance.* Available from http://uhra.herts.ac.uk/dspace/bistream/2299/1979/i/Expert+Patinets+Programme.pdf.

Wilson, P.M., Kendall, S. and Brooks, F. (2006b) Nurses' responses to expert patients. The rhetoric and reality of self-management in long-term conditions: a grounded theory study. *International Journal of Nursing Studies* 43(7): 803–18.

Wiltshire Primary Care Trust (2007) *Step by Step: Reforming Community Service in Wiltshire.* Available from http://www.wiltshirepct.nhs.uk/ReformingCommunityServices/RCSStepbyStepJune_Issue2.pdf.

World Health Organization (2008) Information Technology in Support of Health Care. Available from http://www.who.int/eht/en/InformationTech.pdf.

Youngson, R. (2008) *Compassion in Healthcare: The Missing Dimension of Healthcare Reform?* Delivery the Future Today. Available from http://www.debatepapers.org.uk.

Useful websites

Care Service Improvement Partnership: http://www.networks.csip.org.uk/telecarefactsheets; http://www.networks.csip.org.uk/telecarenewsletters; http://www.networks.csip.org.uk/telecareservices; http://www.networks.csip.org.uk/telecareoutcomes

Connecting for Health: http://www.connectingforhealth.nhs.uk/

Expert Patients Programme Community Interest Company: http://www. expertpatients.co.uk/public/default.aspx.

Hope for Tomorrow: http://www.hopefortomorrow.org.uk

Partnership for Older People Project: http://www.cat.csip.org.uk/index.cfm?pid= 625

Self Care for Primary Care: http://www.selfcareconnect.co.uk

Telecare Aware: http://www.telecareaware.com

Torbay Care Trust: http://www.torbaycaretrust.nhs.uk/

West Lothian Community Health and Care Partnership: http://www. westlothianchcp.org.uk/ese

Whole System Demonstrators Network: http://www.wsdactionnetwork.org.uk/ about_wsdan/

Index